emergencycare

A SELF-ASSESSMENT
GUIDE

Tim Hodgetts

MB BS(Hons), MRCP(UK), FFAEM, DipIMC RCSEd, RAMC
Consultant and Specialty Adviser in Accident and Emergency Medicine,
Frimley Park Hospital, Camberley

Ian Greaves

MB ChB, MRCP(UK), DTM&H, DipIMC RCSEd
Registrar in Accident and Emergency Medicine,
St James' University Hospital, Leeds

Keith Porter

MB BS, FRCS, DipIMC RCSEd
Consultant Trauma Surgeon,
Selly Oak Hospital, Birmingham

WB Saunders
London · Philadelphia · Toronto · Tokyo

WB Saunders Company Ltd 24-28 Oval Road
London NW1 7DX

The Curtis Center
Independence Square West
Philadelphia, PA 19106-3399, USA

Harcourt Brace & Company
55 Horner Avenue
Toronto, Ontario M8Z 4X6, Canada

Harcourt Brace & Company, Australia
30–52 Smidmore Street
Marrickville, NSW 2204, Australia

Harcourt Brace & Company, Japan
Ichibancho Central Building, 22-1 Ichibancho
Chiyoda-ku, Tokyo 102, Japan

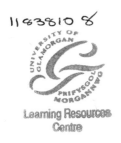

A catalogue record for this book is available from the British Library

ISBN 0-7020-2345-0

Typeset by LaserScript, Mitcham, Surrey
Printed in Great Britain by WBC Book Manufacturers, Bridgend, Mid-Glamorgan

CONTENTS

HOW TO USE THIS BOOK

This book is designed to be used as an adjunct to *Emergency Care: A Textbook for Paramedics*.

The book is divided into twenty papers, which cover the same topics as the textbook in the same order. After reading the associated chapter(s) in the textbook, it is then possible to test your knowledge and understanding by doing the corresponding 'paper'. The book may also be used as a stand-alone self-assessment text for paramedical, medical and nursing personnel involved in the delivery of pre-hospital emergency care.

Each paper follows a similar format with:

- Multiple choice questions
- Short answer questions
- A picture quiz
- Case histories

A general 'test paper' is also included.

Tim Hodgetts
Ian Greaves
Keith Porter

SCENE APPROACH AND ASSESSMENT

Refer to Chapter 1 of
Emergency Care: A Textbook for Paramedics

MULTIPLE CHOICE

1.1 When driving to the scene:

A. The priority is to reach the scene as fast as possible

B. Blue lights give a legal right of way

C. Defensive driving involves keeping a safe distance from the vehicle in front

D. The *two-second rule* refers to the safe time between two moving vehicles

E. A siren is a poor advanced warning device on the motorway

1.2 The following are true of personal protective equipment:

A. A visor provides *primary* eye protection

B. Latex gloves protect against contamination from the patient

C. Overalls *must have* high visibility bands

D. Footwear *must be* oil and acid resistant

E. A jacket protects against direct flame

1.3 **You are the first emergency service vehicle to attend the scene of a road traffic accident with three persons trapped and seriously injured. Your priorities include:**

1. Taking control of the situation

2. Treating the casualties

3. Sorting the casualties into priorities for treatment

4. Requesting further assistance

5. Parking to protect the scene

The order in which you should perform these actions is:

A. 1–2–3–4–5

B. 5–1–4–3–2

C. 1–5–4–3–2

D. 5–1–3–4–2

E. 5–1–3–2–4

1.4 **The following injuries to the driver would be anticipated from a driver's side-on impact:**

A. Ipsilateral* pelvis fracture

B. Contralateral[†] femur fracture

C. Liver injury

D. Foot entrapped by pedals

E. Laceration above left eye from rear-view mirror

*Ipsilateral = same side
[†]Contralateral = opposite side

1.5 **The mnemonic 'ETHANE' reminds the paramedic of the important information to pass to control following an initial assessment. This information includes:**

A. Your location

B. The vital signs of the casualties

C. The emergency services present at the scene

D. The potential hazards

E. The access to the scene

SHORT ANSWERS

1.6 Define *defensive driving*. List the defensive driving techniques.

1.7 List the privileges afforded by a 'blue light'. Who is legally responsible should you hit another vehicle when you go through a red traffic light?

PICTURE QUIZ

1.8 Where would you park the first ambulance at the scene, and why?

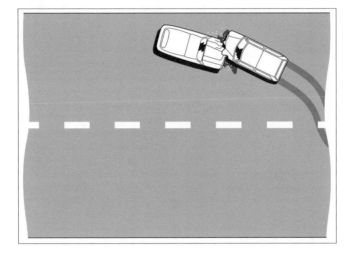

1.9 **What injuries would you anticipate in the driver of this vehicle?**

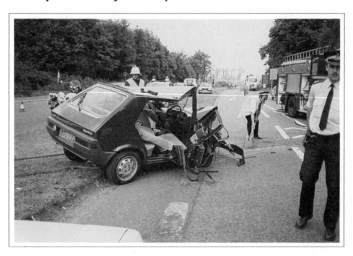

1.10 **What hazards are present to yourself and the casualties at this incident?**

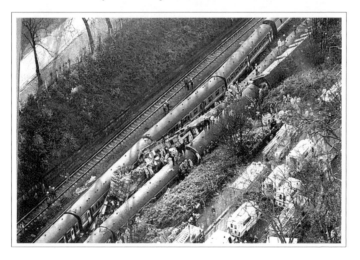

SCENE APPROACH AND ASSESSMENT

MULTIPLE CHOICE

1.1 (A) F (B) F (C) T (D) T (E) T

When driving to the scene the priority is safety, not speed. A blue light confers no legal right of way: it is the courtesy of other road users that allows the emergency service vehicle to pass. Defensive driving involves keeping a safe distance between your vehicle and the vehicle in front. When driving on a motorway there should be two seconds of distance between vehicles – remember, *only a fool breaks the two second rule*. A siren gives poor advanced warning of an approaching emergency service vehicle on a motorway. In this situation intermittent dipped and full-beam headlights are particularly effective.

1.2 (A) F (B) T (C) T (D) F (E) F

A visor provides primary face protection and secondary eye protection (dust can still get into the eyes under the visor). Primary eye protection is provided by goggles or safety glasses. Latex gloves will protect against patient contamination, particularly blood, and reduce the risk of cross-infection with HIV, hepatitis B, and hepatitis C viruses. In the pre-hospital setting, these gloves can easily be damaged; heavy-duty gloves may also be appropriate during the patient access phase of the rescue.

Overalls should be of high visibility, with reflective strips, and should be marked 'PARAMEDIC' or 'TECHNICIAN'. Additionally, they may be fire retardant. Jackets should also be of high visibility, and bear appropriate markings. Oil- and acid-resistant boots would be ideal for an industrial or transport accident, but are unlikely to be suitable day-to-day footwear for the majority of jobs.

1.3   5–1–4–3–2 = B

The priorities at the scene of a road traffic accident can be remembered as **CONTROL, then ACT**.

First park to protect the incident, 'on-line' on a motorway or dual carriageway, or in the 'fend-off' on a single carriageway road. Take **CONTROL** of the situation. (This will be implicit by your arrival in an emergency service vehicle, but you may wish to ask bystander(s) explicitly to perform a number of tasks.) Make an assessment of the situation, including hazards and the number and severity of casualties (**A**CT). Communicate with ambulance control, passing the information about your assessment (see question 1.5) and requesting appropriate support (**A**CT). Finally sort, or 'triage', the three casualties into priorities for treatment and transport, and provide life-saving treatment at the scene and *en route* to hospital (AC**T**).

1.4   (A) T (B) F (C) T (D) F (E) F

Characteristic injuries from a side impact on the driver's side will include:

- right-sided head injury
- right-sided arm injury (fractured humerus)
- right-sided chest injury (flail chest; pulmonary contusion)
- right-sided abdominal injury (liver)
- right-sided pelvic injury
- right-sided leg injury (fracture of the femur; fracture of the tibia and fibula)

Foot entrapment from the pedals would tend to occur when the floor pan buckles in a head-on collision. A laceration from the rear view mirror above the left eye is a characteristic driver's injury in a head-on collision.

1.5   (A) T (B) F (C) T (D) T (E) T

The mnemonic to remember the initial information to pass on from the scene is **'ETHANE'**:

E	Exact location
T	Type of incident
H	Hazards, present and potential
A	Access to the scene
N	Number and severity of casualties
E	Emergency services, present and required

A 'present' hazard would be petrol, but its 'potential' is fire. Vital signs of patients or exact details on the nature of injuries would not be given at this stage.

SHORT ANSWERS

1.6 Defensive driving is the technique of advanced driving taught to emergency service personnel. It involves maximizing the capabilities of the vehicle while driving safely and responsibly at all times. Techniques include:

- Retaining a safe distance between your vehicle and the vehicle in front when travelling at speed
- Adjusting your speed so that you can always stop in the distance that can be seen (for example, on a winding road)
- Leaving enough room for manoeuvring between your vehicle and the vehicle in front when travelling in heavy traffic
- Treating a 'stop' sign or red traffic light with caution, and giving way if necessary to the traffic that has priority
- Constantly observing the road ahead and anticipating the hazards. (A parked car with brake lights on is not a hazard, but as soon as the brake lights extinguish, the car may either pull out, or the door open.)

1.7 There are no legal privileges of a blue light, although it is accepted that an ambulance, police, or fire service vehicle responding to an emergency will exceed the speed limit, and may treat a red traffic light as a 'give way'. Should any accident occur during the infringement of traffic regulations, then it is the responsibility of the emergency service driver. An ambulance driver who causes such an accident can expect to be prosecuted for dangerous driving.

This is not the situation world-wide. In Germany, it is the responsibility of the ordinary road user to make way for an emergency service vehicle which has its beacons/siren engaged. An accident in these circumstances is invariably judged as the responsibility of the ordinary road user.

PICTURE QUIZ

1.8   The position for an ambulance to park is shown in the figure below.

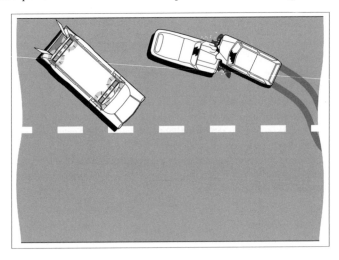

1.9   The injuries anticipated from a head-on collision are:

- Head and scalp injury, with possible depression of conscious level
- Facial fractures (windscreen/steering wheel), with possible airway compromise
- Cervical spine flexion–extension injury
- Chest injury (sternal flail; pulmonary contusion; fractured ribs; pneumothorax)
- Seatbelt tension injury (fractured clavicle; abdominal viscus perforation)
- Abdominal compression from steering column (viscus perforation; ruptured hemi-diaphragm)
- Upper-limb indirect force injury (scaphoid fracture; Colles' fracture; radial head fracture; elbow or shoulder dislocation)
- Patella fracture, and/or femoral shaft fracture, and/or posterior dislocation of the hip (dashboard and engine compartment intrusion)
- Lower tibia/ankle fracture–dislocation (buckling floor pan)

1.10   The hazards at this type of incident include:

Elements	Rain, cold, wind, sun
Rail	Downed power lines or live rail; diesel trains even when the power source is isolated
Wreckage	Glass, sharp metal, fire and smoke
Goods	Possible chemical hazard
Patients	Blood; sharps following interventions

PATIENT ASSESSMENT

Refer to Chapter 2 of
Emergency Care: A Textbook for Paramedics

MULTIPLE CHOICE

2.1   Predictors of serious injury include:

A.   Ejection from a vehicle

B.   Post-traumatic amnesia

C.   A fall from more than 5 metres

D.   A fall from a horse

E.   Death of another occupant of the vehicle

2.2   The following are true:

A.   The first priority at any scene is the *airway*

B.   Vehicle entrapment equates with more serious injury

C.   The elderly are more at risk of serious injury following any trauma

D.   Children are more at risk than adults of serious injury following blunt trauma

E.   A detectable radial pulse in an adult equates with a minimum systolic blood pressure of 100 mmHg

2.3   In pre-hospital care the primary survey:

A.   Is not relevant in medical illness

B.   Is followed by resuscitation

C.   Must be followed by complete exposure of the patient

D.   Includes an assessment of the patient's neurological status

E.   Includes immobilization of the cervical spine

2.4 **Normal values in an adult include:**

A. A capillary refill time of less than 2 seconds

B. A respiratory rate of 12–18 per minute

C. A pulse oximetry reading of >96% on air

D. A blood pressure of 95/60 mmHg

E. A blood glucose test strip of 2.0 mmol/l

2.5 **Concerning the mini-neurological examination:**

A. AVPU has no correlation with GCS

B. Glasgow Coma Scale is assessed in the primary survey

C. An assessment of the pupillary size and reaction is included

D. 'U' stands for 'unconscious'

E. There is an assessment for lateralizing limb signs

2.6 **The following will first be noted in the secondary survey:**

A. Bleeding from the ears

B. Compound fracture of the femur

C. Abdominal tenderness

D. Spinal deformity

E. Rectal bleeding

2.7 **A 35-year-old male who has been involved in a road traffic accident and has sustained an obvious compound fracture of the right femoral shaft becomes less responsive on loading into the ambulance. Your first priority is to:**

A. Transfer rapidly to hospital

B. Reassess the airway

C. Administer intravenous fluids

D. Check the blood glucose

E. Increase the oxygen therapy

2.8 **An increased respiratory rate may be a sign of:**

A.   Hypovolaemia

B.   Anxiety

C.   Partially obstructed airway

D.   Diaphragmatic rupture

E.   Hypothermia

SHORT ANSWERS

2.9 You attend an elderly lady in the street who has an obvious fractured neck of femur following a slip on the ice. Why should you undertake a primary survey?

2.10 List the essential elements of a medical history.

PICTURE QUIZ

2.11 What are the priorities in this patient?

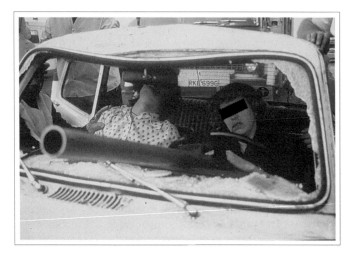

PATIENT ASSESSMENT

MULTIPLE CHOICE

2.1 (A) T (B) F (C) T (D) T (E) T

Ejection from a vehicle is invariably associated with a high-energy transfer from:

- Ground impact
- Vehicular impact and intrusion
- The process of ejection

Post-traumatic amnesia may be associated with minor head injury as well as severe injury. Typically, in a simple concussion the patient can remember the accident being about to happen, but loses a few seconds of memory after the accident.

Statistically, serious and life-threatening injuries are more likely in falls over 5 metres, but someone landing on their head at 3 metres is probably more serious than landing on their feet at 5 metres – so apply common sense.

Falls from a horse are often associated with crush injuries as the horse rolls over the rider. There is also a high incidence of spinal injury in these patients.

Death of another car occupant highlights the magnitude of energy transfer, and the possibility of serious injury to the surviving occupant. Even when there is no obvious injury and physiological signs are normal, people in this group should always be taken to hospital.

2.2 (A) F (B) T (C) T (D) T (E) F

The first priority at any scene is *safety*: yourself, the scene, and the casualties in that order. Airway is the first prioirity in the primary survey.

Most vehicular accidents do not involve entrapment. When it does occur entrapment may be *relative* (the occupant is injured and cannot open the door, for example, because of a broken arm), or *absolute* (the occupant is physically restrained by the deformed wreckage). Entrapments are invariably associated with higher energy impacts and, therefore, with more serious injury.

The elderly, because of the general frailty of their skeletons and the likelihood of pre-existing disease, are more at risk of serious injury following any trauma. An example is a trip on a paving stone causing a fractured neck of femur.

Children have elastic skeletons and, particularly in the chest, blunt energy is not absorbed by the skeleton to the same extent as adults (leaving the underlying organs more vulnerable). In addition, because of a child's relative short stature, an injury which may produce a fracture of the tibia or femur in an adult, for example, a pedestrian collison with the front of a car, may produce a major cavity injury (abdomen or chest) in a child.

Assessment of the carotid, femoral and radial pulses allows a rough determination of systolic blood pressure (carotid present = >60 mmHg; femoral = >70 mmHg; radial = >80 mmHg).

2.3   (A) F (B) F (C) F (D) T (E) T

A primary survey forms the basis of clinical assessment in medical illness and injury, with the assessment of airway, breathing, circulation, disability and appropriate exposure. Any life-threatening problem identified during the primary survey is immediately treated. The primary survey and resuscitation, therefore, occur simultaneously. A patient's neurological status is assessed using the AVPU scale (see question 2.5). The cervical spine is stabilized in conjunction with airway assessment.

2.4   (A) T (B) T (C) T (D) F (E) F

Pressure on the capillary bed for 5 seconds produces blanching, and this should refill to normal colour within 2 seconds. This *capillary refill test* is an indication of peripheral perfusion, and is prolonged in the hypovolaemic patient. It is also prolonged in the cold, although in these circumstances it can be crudely equated with the paramedic's own capillary refill. It cannot be assessed in the dark.

A patient with a respiratory rate of less than 12 and greater than 18 requires supplemental oxygen. If the rate is less than 10 or more than 29, then consideration should be given to supportive ventilation.

The normal pulse oximeter reading on air at sea level in a fit adult is over 96%. Importantly, supplemental oxygen may maintain the oxygen saturation and give a 'normal' reading even in the presence of hypoventilation and significant carbon dioxide retention.

The normal blood glucose level is 4–6 mmol/l.

2.5 (A) F (B) F (C) T (D) F (E) F

AVPU forms part of the mini-neurological examination in the primary survey. It can be correlated roughly with the Glasgow Coma Scale (GCS).

A	Alert	GCS 15
V	Responds to voice	GCS 13
P	Responds to pain	GCS 8
U	Unresponsive	GCS 3

As the primary survey is a rapid initial assessment, the mini-neurological examination is restricted to *AVPU + pupillary reaction to light*. An assessment of lateralizing signs is not made. The GCS is formally measured in the secondary survey. The **best** response is recorded, if the response differs in the limbs. In critical trauma, there may not be time to perform a secondary survey, and therefore a GCS, before arrival in hospital.

2.6 (A) T (B) F (C) T (D) T (E) T

In time-critical trauma it may only be possible to undertake a primary survey pre-hospital. Bleeding from the ears is likely to be detected during a detailed examination of the head, and indicates a compound middle cranial fossa fracture (basal skull fracture). A compound fracture of the femur would almost certainly be noted in the primary survey when an assessment is made for obvious external blood loss.

Spinal deformity is noted when the patient is log-rolled in a controlled manner, and the spine systematically inspected and palpated. Unless rectal bleeding is catastrophic, it would go unrecognized until a rectal examination is performed in hospital (often in conjunction with the log-roll).

2.7 (A) F (B) T (C) F (D) F (E) F

Whenever a patient deteriorates, it is essential to return to the ABC assessment. In this case it would be important to ensure a clear airway, to give high-flow oxygen, to exclude a life-threatening treatable chest condition and to arrest external haemorrhage. Intravenous volume replacement can be started on the rapid journey to hospital, and it would be important to advise the hospital of your impending arrival.

2.8 (A) T (B) T (C) T (D) T (E) F

Hypovolaemia results in decreased delivery of oxygen to the tissues and this is compensated for in part by a rise in the respiratory rate.

Anxiety by itself will generate an increased respiratory rate, and partial airway obstruction will cause stimulation of the respiratory centre from hypoxia. *Hyperthermia* will raise the respiratory rate, but it will progressively slow with hypothermia.

SHORT ANSWERS

2.9 Whilst this could be an injury in isolation, it may be associated with other injuries, some of which may be life-threatening. For this reason, each patient is approached systematically, and a primary survey performed.

Approximately 5% of all patients with femoral neck fractures have other injuries, commonly including a Colles' fracture ('dinner fork' deformity of the wrist) or a fracture of the neck of the humerus sustained by partially falling on to an outstretched hand. It is also important to ask yourself 'What is the cause of the fall?' It could be precipitated by a myocardial infarction, epileptic fit or hypoglycaemia.

2.10 The components of a medical history can be remembered with the mnemonic *AMPLE*:

A	Allergies
M	Medicines
P	Past medical history
L	Last food and drink
E	Events leading up to the current problem

It is important to establish if the patient has any allergies before administering drugs, with the exception of a cardiac arrest. Medication may influence the response to illness or injury (patients on beta-blockers will not get a tachycardia with hypovolaemia) or may interact with further medication given as emergency treatment. Past medical history may give you the diagnosis, if the problem is recurrent. Knowing the time of last food and drink may influence the timing of an emergency operation.

PICTURE QUIZ

2.11 **The first priority is *safety*:**
- Yourself
- The scene
- The casualty

Priorities of care are:

- Airway with control of the cervical spine
- Breathing with oxygen
- Circulation with control of external bleeding
- Disability assessment (AVPU + pupils)
- Exposure limited to that which is essential, while aware of the risks of the environment (hypothermia, elements)

The orthopaedic injury will be treated following a limited secondary survey. This will include wound dressing and leg splintage. All trauma patients require oxygen. An intravenous infusion should be considered if there is a long transport time to hospital. Analgesia is important and could include a combination of reassurance, splintage, Entonox and intravenous analgesic (e.g. nalbuphine).

BASIC LIFE SUPPORT

Refer to Chapter 3 of
Emergency Care: A Textbook for Paramedics

MULTIPLE CHOICE

3.1   In adult basic life support with two rescuers:

A.   The compression to ventilation ratio is 15:2

B.   A handkerchief may be used to improve hygiene

C.   A precordial thump should be performed

D.   Normal compression depth is 3 cm

E.   Each ventilation cycle should take 4 seconds

3.2   The Heimlich manoeuvre:

A.   Is recommended for children over 1 year old

B.   Is safe for the pregnant patient

C.   Is better than back blows

D.   Is contraindicated in the conscious patient

E.   Should be attempted a maximum of five times

3.3   External cardiac compression:

A.   If performed competently, will produce up to 60% of normal cardiac output

B.   Is more haemodynamically efficient than open cardiac massage

C.   Should be performed approximately 120 times per minute in adults

D.   Is performed using the heel of the hand over the lower sternum

E.   Produces blood flow owing to direct compression of the heart

3.4   Concerning the adult in respiratory arrest:

A.   The carotid pulse should be taken for 15 seconds

B.   Opiate abuse is a common cause

C.   Five rescue breaths are given

D.   Cardiac arrest will follow without appropriate intervention

E.   The diagnosis is established by 'look, listen and feel' for 10 seconds

3.5   Common causes of inadequate ventilation include:

A.   Gastric distension following overinflation

B.   Airway obstruction owing to a foreign body

C.   Failure to pinch the patient's nose

D.   Asynchronous ventilation and cardiac compression

E.   Incorrect simple airway manoeuvres

3.6   Basic life support:

A.   Includes the use of oral or nasal airways

B.   Produces a return to spontaneous circulation in 5% of cases

C.   May be abandoned after 1 hour in all patients

D.   Carries a significant risk of rescuer infection with HIV

E.   May be effective in relieving an obstructed airway

3.7   Concerning the airway:

A.   A finger sweep may worsen airway obstruction

B.   Chin-lift is contraindicated when cervical spine injury is suspected

C.   Well-fitting false teeth should be left in place

D.   The *triple airway manoeuvre* is head tilt + chin lift + jaw thrust

E.   Care of the airway is the first priority with a collapsed patient

SHORT ANSWERS

3.8   What is the 'SAFE approach'?

3.9   List the causes of ineffective chest compression.

3.10   Describe the simple airway manoeuvres.

3.11   What is the emergency treatment of a choking adult?

PICTURE QUIZ

3.12   It is safe to approach this patient, but you have no further information. What are your priorities?

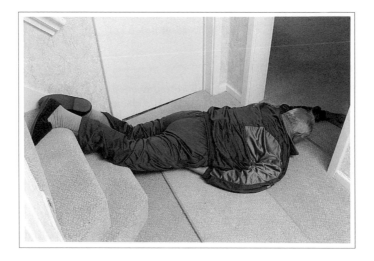

BASIC LIFE SUPPORT

MULTIPLE CHOICE

3.1   (A) F (B) F (C) F (D) F (E) T

With two rescuers, the compression to ventilation ratio is 5:1 (15:2 with a single rescuer). The use of a handkerchief, although perhaps aesthetically more acceptable than mouth-to-mouth, will not improve hygiene, and conversely by trapping bacteria and debris it may increase the likelihood of patient infection. A simple 'foil' device (plastic sheet with bite guard) may be used. The precordial thump is not part of the current (European Resuscitation Council, 1992) basic life support guidelines. The normal sternal compression depth in an adult is 4–5 cm.

3.2   (A) F (B) F (C) F (D) F (E) F

The Heimlich manoeuvre is only recommended for children over the age of 5 years, because of the potential risk of damage to intra-abdominal organs. It is not recommended for use in pregnant patients. There is no limit to how many times it can be attempted, but it is recommended to alternate with back blows. Back blows are equally as effective and are often attempted first, but there is no scientific reason for this.

3.3   (A) F (B) F (C) F (D) T (E) T

The best external (closed) chest compression technique will produce only 30% of normal cardiac output; open cardiac compressions will produce up to 50% of normal output. The mechanism for the pump effect with closed chest compressions is a combination of direct cardiac compression and an indirect increase in intrathoracic pressure. In an adult, the objective is to maintain a rate of 80 compressions per minute.

3.4 (A) F (B) T (C) F (D) T (E) T

The presence or absence of breathing or a central pulse is established in each case by a check lasting for up to 10 seconds. Opiate abuse is an increasingly common cause of respiratory arrest. Ten rescue breaths are given to the victim of a respiratory arrest (no breathing, but pulse present) by a single rescuer before leaving the casualty to call for help. Hypoxic cardiac arrest will inevitably follow respiratory arrest unless artificial ventilation is started.

3.5 (A) T (B) T (C) T (D) F (E) T

Asynchronous ventilation and chest compression may improve the effectiveness of ventilation.

3.6 (A) F (B) F (C) F (D) F (E) T

Traditionally basic life support (BLS) has meant the support of 'ABC' without the use of equipment, but this definition has been extended to include the use of a foil (face shield) or pocket mask. BLS will not result in the return of spontaneous circulation – it is a holding procedure until advanced life support can be started. This is true unless the original diagnosis of cardiorespiratory arrest was erroneous. Occasionally, BLS may relieve an obstructed airway either as air is forced past the obstruction or when chest compressions cause the obstruction to be expelled. Prolonged BLS is appropriate in victims of hypothermia and especially children.

3.7 (A) T (B) F (C) T (D) F (E) F

Careless use of the finger sweep may cause a foreign body to impact further down the airway, worsening a partial obstruction or rendering it complete. Head tilt is not recommended in suspected cervical spine injury, when jaw thrust or chin lift should be used. The *triple airway manoeuvre* is head tilt + chin lift + mouth open. The first priority at the scene of a collapsed patient is *SAFETY*.

SHORT ANSWERS

3.8 The *SAFE approach* is:

S Shout for help
A Approach with care
F Free from danger
E Evaluate

- Airway
- Breathing
- Circulation

3.9 The causes of ineffective chest compression are:

1. Wrong hand position:
   - Too high – the heart is not effectively compressed
   - Too low – the stomach is compressed increasing the risk of aspiration
   - Too lateral – this is ineffective and the underlying organs may be damaged

2. Overenthusiastic effort:
   - Causes cardiac damage
   - Fractures ribs, causing damage to underlying organs (liver, spleen)

3. Inadequate effort:
   - May result from poor positioning and failure to use weight of rescuer's body during compression
   - May result from fatigue of prolonged resuscitation

4. Failure to release between compressions:
   - Prevents venous return and filling of the heart

5. Inadequate or excessive rate:
   - Optimum is ~80 per minute in adults and 100 per minute in children

3.10 The simple airway manoeuvres are:

1. Removal of obstruction. This is by finger sweep (blind finger sweeps are not recommended, as they may further impact a foreign body), suction (hand-held, foot operated or battery operated), or under direct vision using a laryngoscope and Magill's forceps.

2. Triple airway manoeuvre. This is a combination of head tilt + chin lift + mouth open. It is a suitable manoeuvre for basic life support, although is not the generally recommended manouevre to open the airway following trauma, because of the potential to compromise a cervical spine injury. However, the airway is *always* more important than the cervical spine and, if this manoeuvre is required to open the airway following trauma, then this is acceptable.

3. Jaw thrust. This is the preferred airway opening manoeuvre in the trauma victim, and can be performed while simultaneously providing manual stabilization of the cervical spine. As the tongue is attached to the floor of the mouth, the tongue is lifted away from the pharynx as the jaw is pushed forwards.

3.11 Choking is usually caused by an attempt to talk and breathe at the same time, with a mouth full of food. The following algorithm can be followed:

Victim responsive

Reassure and tell the victim to try to cough, while bending forwards

↓

5 × back blows

↓

5 × Heimlich manoeuvres

↓

Repeat cycles of back blows and Heimlich manoeuvres until foreign body is dislodged or patient becomes unresponsive

Victim unresponsive

Open airway

↓

Hook out visible foreign body

↓

Attempt to ventilate

↓

5 × abdominal thrusts astride the patient

↓

5 × back blows

↓

Return to step 1, open the airway and repeat sequence

↓

Move rapidly to surgical airway if these manoeuvres are ineffective

---

PICTURE QUIZ

3.12 Your initial priority is always *safety* – yourself, the scene and the casualty. As you approach you will 'read' the scene and start to fit the puzzle together. Did this man fall down the stairs, or did he collapse from a medical condition and the fall was secondary? Is there any history immediately available? ('Thank God you're here! He said he had chest pain going up the stairs then suddenly collapsed!')

Open and clear the airway, while maintaining cervical spine control. Jaw thrust would be the most appropriate manoeuvre. Assess for breathing. Feel for a central pulse. If there is cardiac arrest, start basic life support, while your colleague prepares to monitor the cardiac rhythm through the paddles of a manual defibrillator, or through the large chest electrodes of the semi-automatic (advisory) defibrillator.

If basic life support needs to be continued in transit to hospital, it would be best for the patient to be evacuated on a spinal board because of the risk of associated injury in the fall. If the cardiac rhythm is electro-mechanical dissociation, treatable traumatic causes should be considered and treated early (hypovolaemia, tension pneumothorax).

AIRWAY AND INTRAVENOUS ACCESS

Refer to Chapters 4, 5 and 6 of
Emergency Care: A Textbook for Paramedics

MULTIPLE CHOICE

4.1 **The following are indications for intubation pre-hospital:**

A. Cardiorespiratory arrest

B. Flail chest

C. All patients with a Glasgow Coma Scale of <9

D. All patients who tolerate a Guedel airway

E. All victims of smoke inhalation

4.2 **Concerning orotracheal intubation:**

A. Intubation of a single main bronchus may occur

B. Tension pneumothorax may be precipitated in the presence of chest injury

C. Oesophageal intubation may be detected by end-tidal CO_2 monitoring

D. For air transportation, the cuff should be filled with water

E. It is contraindicated in cervical spine injury

4.3 **The following relate to the anatomy of the paediatric airway:**

A. The airway is narrowest at the level of the cricoid in children

B. The larynx is relatively more posterior in neonates

C. The infant's head is proportionally larger than the adult head

D. The diameter of the neonate's trachea is 2.0–3.0 mm

E. Infants under 3 months are obligatory nasal breathers

4.4 Concerning the airway:

A. Attempts at intubation can produce laryngospasm

B. A finger sweep is recommended to remove an upper airway foreign body in a child

C. Uncuffed endotracheal tubes are used up to the age of 10 years

D. Central cyanosis occurs earlier in children than in adults

E. The epiglottis in a child is relatively smaller than in an adult

4.5 With regard to respiratory control:

A. A fall in PCO_2 stimulates respiration

B. A fall in blood pH stimulates respiration

C. High concentration oxygen should be given in a patient with chronic obstructive pulmonary disease following severe trauma

D. The phrenic nerve is supplied by C4, C5 and C6 nerve roots

E. Opiates suppress respiration by affecting chemoreceptors in the lungs

4.6 Concerning abnormal respiratory noises:

A. Noisy breathing during inspiration is common in asthma

B. Stridor may be due to partial obstruction from a foreign body

C. Epiglottitis commonly produces marked stridor

D. An expiratory wheeze suggests obstruction at or below the larynx

E. Wheezes may occur in left ventricular failure

4.7 The causes of hypoventilation include:

A. Myocardial infarction

B. Diabetes mellitus

C. Head injury

D. Myasthenia gravis

E. Electrocution

4.8   Tachypnoea characteristically occurs in:

A.   Hyperglycaemic diabetic coma

B.   High cervical cord injuries

C.   Haemothorax

D.   Aspirin overdose

E.   Pregnancy

4.9   Relating to endotracheal tubes:

A.   A 9.0 mm internal diameter is the 'universal' adult size

B.   The tube length is twice the distance from the corner of the mouth to the angle of the jaw

C.   The correct internal diameter for a child is [age ÷ 4] + 2

D.   In adults the cuff should be deflated every 20 minutes to prevent damage to the trachea

E.   Children do not require a cuffed tube because the incidence of regurgitation is much lower

4.10   Oxygen therapy:

A.   Should be given to all victims of significant trauma

B.   Should be given at a rate of 10–15 L/min

C.   Can mask alveolar hypoventilation

D.   Can only be given at 100% via an endotracheal tube

E.   From a 'D'-sized cylinder will last for 45 minutes at 15 L/min

4.11   The oropharyngeal (Guedel) airway:

A.   Is sized from the corner of the mouth to the earlobe

B.   Is inserted concave downwards in children

C.   Can precipitate vomiting

D.   Should be inserted with a mouth gag when the teeth are clenched

E.   If too small, may aggravate the airway obstruction

4.12 The nasopharyngeal airway:

A. Is contraindicated in the head-injured patient

B. Position is checked using a laryngoscope

C. Size required will approximate to the diameter of the patient's ring finger

D. Is secured to the nose with a safety pin

E. Is generally not used in children

4.13 Where there is a risk of cervical spine injury:

A. The triple airway manoeuvre is recommended

B. Cervical traction is maintained manually until the application of a semi-rigid collar

C. Cervical spine protection has overall priority

D. The semi-rigid collar should not be removed during intubation

E. The agitated patient should be physically restrained

4.14 The following statements regarding fluid resuscitation are true:

A. All shocked patients should receive colloid

B. Haemaccel® has a shelf life of 1 year

C. Three times the volume of colloid compared to crystalloid is required to achieve the same effect

D. A colloid is a suspension of particles

E. Resuscitation with normal saline alone in large volumes may produce an acidosis

4.15 The flow through a cannula is:

A. Reduced in cold weather

B. Most importantly determined by the diameter

C. Proportional to the length

D. The same for colloids and crystalloids

E. Reduced at altitude

4.16 **Regarding intraosseous infusion:**

A. Fluid may be infused satisfactorily under its own pressure

B. It can only be used in one site

C. It is contraindicated in children with brittle bone disease

D. The leg should be protected in a box splint

E. Should not be used in children over age 6 years

4.17 **Laryngeal mask airway:**

A. Cannot be used in children

B. If correctly placed will prevent gastric aspiration

C. Requires insertion under direct vision using a laryngoscope

D. Is also known as the PTLA or 'Combi-Tube'

E. Has been proven to be a useful alternative in resuscitation during cardiac arrest

SHORT ANSWERS

4.18 List the causes of airway obstruction.

4.19 What are the alternatives to endotracheal intubation?

4.20 You are called to a house fire where the Fire Service has just rescued a 25-year-old student who is unconscious, has a respiratory rate of 8 per minute, and has soot around his mouth and nostrils. List your actions and monitoring on the way to hospital.

PICTURE QUIZ

4.21 What is this equipment for? Describe the procedure.

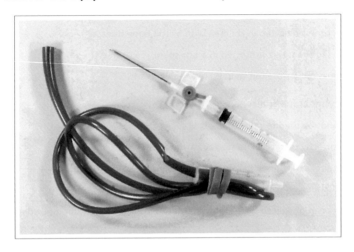

AIRWAY AND INTRAVENOUS ACCESS

MULTIPLE CHOICE

4.1 (A) T (B) F (C) F (D) F (E) F

The management of cardiac arrest should follow the current European Resuscitation Council guidelines, and the exact timing of intubation in the protocol is dependent upon the cardiac arrest rhythm.

Most patients with flail chest will benefit from simple manual stabilization, and do not require intubation for this injury in isolation in the pre-hospital setting.

Patients who are deeply unconscious (Glasgow Come Scale of 8 or less – the definition of 'coma') would ideally require intubation to protect the airway, and this may be influenced by the transit time to hospital. However, unless the patient is totally unresponsive (GCS 3), the presence of a gag reflex will mean that the patient cannot be safely intubated without pharmacological agents (anaesthesia and muscle relaxant). In this case, airway and ventilation is maintained by an oro- or naso-pharyngeal adjunct, and a bag-valve-mask device. Patients may tolerate an oropharyngeal airway with a GCS of greater than 3, so this cannot be used as a clear indication for intubation.

A patient who has smoke inhalation and evidence of airway burn with stridor requires rapid transport to hospital. Intubation under these circumstances is very difficult, even in the most expert anaesthetist's hands, and it may be necessary to resort to a surgical airway.

4.2 (A) T (B) T (C) T (D) T (E) F

If the endotracheal tube is too long, then intubation of a main bronchus is a common problem, usually down the right side because the bronchus branches from the trachea at a more oblique angle. Listening to both sides of the chest post-intubation is mandatory. In chest injury, positive pressure ventilation, achieved via orotracheal intubation, may produce an air leak through damaged lung parenchyma and a tension pneumothorax.

Intubation of the oesophagus is a potentially fatal complication. It is not negligent to intubate the oesophagus, only to fail to recognize the complication. End-tidal CO_2 monitoring may assist in differentiating between oesophageal and tracheal intubation: tracheal air has a high carbon dioxide content, stomach air does not.

For helicopter transportation in the United Kingdom, changes in altitude are unlikely to result in significant changes in air pressure and relative inflation of an endotracheal tube cuff. For high altitude fixed-wing transport, filling the cuff with water should be considered. Certain military casevac aircraft can be pressurized to sea level, but this causes significant degradation of the fuselage. Alternatively, military aircraft can literally 'skip the waves'.

The airway takes precedence over the cervical spine, although every attempt is made to maintain spinal stability while maintaining a clear airway. During intubation in-line manual stabilization is provided and the collar removed.

4.3   (A) T (B) F (C) T (D) F (E) T

The airway is narrowest at the level of the cricoid cartilage in children, which explains why an uncuffed tube provides a snug fit. Furthermore, scarring from pressure necrosis from a cuff may produce permanent airway narrowing in a child. In an adult the narrowest part of the airway is the vocal chords.

The larynx is more anterior in children. The epiglottis is large and floppy, and may need to be lifted directly with the laryngoscope blade in order to see the more anterior larynx (hence a straight-bladed laryngoscope is used).

The infant's head is proportionately larger, and in the supine position the neck is forced into flexion by the prominent occiput. This is equivalent to a small pillow under the head. Further neck flexion may obscure a view of the airway.

A neonate's (newborn baby) trachea is 3–4 mm in diameter, and generally accommodates a 3–3.5 mm tube. Small infants are obligatory nose breathers, so nasal obstruction may be life-threatening.

4.4   (A) T (B) F (C) T (D) F (E) F

Airway reflexes are sensitive in children and, in those who are not profoundly unconscious, instrumentation may cause laryngospasm, bronchospasm, bradycardia and even cardiac arrest.

As the shape of the airway is essentially conical, an attempt to remove a foreign body by finger sweep may have the paradoxical effect of wedging the foreign body further down. It may be better to use back blows to dislodge a foreign body, although Magill's forceps can be used to remove it when visible.

Uncuffed tubes are used in children up to the age of 10 years. The smallest cuffed tube is 6.5 mm internal diameter.

Central cyanosis is a late sign in children, and heralds impending cardiac arrest.

4.5   (A) F (B) T (C) T (D) F (E) F

Breathing is usually controlled by the partial pressure of carbon dioxide in arterial blood, $PaCO_2$. Ventilation is stimulated by a fall in blood pH (a rise in the level of blood acidity), which may occur, for example, in hyperglycaemic diabetic coma.

Some patients with chronic obstructive pulmonary disease (COPD) have adapted to a chronically high $PaCO_2$ and the normal ventilatory drive in response to carbon dioxide is replaced by a hypoxic drive dependent on the low partial pressure of oxygen in arterial blood, PaO_2. Theoretically then, high flow oxygen administered following trauma may suppress ventilatory drive. However, carbon dioxide kills slowly whereas lack of oxygen kills quickly. *Give all trauma victims supplemental high-concentration oxygen.*

The phrenic nerve consists of C3, C4 and C5 nerve roots. Spinal cord injuries in adults are commonly at the C5/6 and C6/7 level: some will have diaphragmatic involvement, while others will spare the diaphragm.

Opiates cause respiratory depression by a central effect on the respiratory centre.

4.6   (A) F (B) T (C) F (D) T (E) T

Asthma characteristically produces an expiratory wheeze, which is a musical noise produced when air is expelled through constricted bronchioles (like a reed instrument). Asthma is reversible obstruction of the lower airways. Wheeze may also be heard in left ventricular failure owing to oedema of the lung parenchyma. Stridor is common in partial upper airway obstruction, such as with a foreign body. Acute epiglottitis produces drooling, and is usually silent.

4.7   (A) F (B) F (C) T (D) T (E) T

Myocardial infarction, and the pain and anxiety it generates, may produce a state of hyperventilation. In diabetic hyperglycaemic coma, there is a metabolic acidosis which stimulates respiration (deep sighing breaths, or Kussmaul's respiration). The respiratory centre may also be depressed following electrocution.

Hypoventilation can occur with head injuries, particularly as a reflection of raised intracranial pressure which also produces hypertension and bradycardia. It is important in the head-injured patient to assess both the respiratory rate and the adequacy of each breath. It is not enough to rely on pulse oximetry to warn of respiratory failure, as a patient receiving high-flow oxygen may sustain a pulse oximetry reading of 100% while hypoventilating and retaining carbon dioxide. A high carbon dioxide level will cause secondary brain injury.

Hypoventilation occurs in myasthenia gravis as a result of respiratory muscle failure.

4.8   (A) T (B) F (C) T (D) T (E) F

Hyperglycaemic diabetic coma produces a metabolic acidosis, which stimulates the respiratory centre. One of the early signs of significant aspirin overdose is tachypnoea, again because of metabolic changes.

With a haemothorax the respiratory rate will rise because of a combination of ventilatory compromise and hypovolaemia. Physiological changes in pregnancy include an increase in the tidal volume and an increase in the minute volume. There is no increase in the respiratory rate.

High cervical cord injuries (above C3) produce immediate apnoea, because of the loss of the function of the phrenic nerve (*C3,4,5 – keeps the diaphragm alive*) and the intercostal muscles. Survival is only possible with immediate respiratory support.

4.9   (A) F (B) T (C) F (D) F (E) F

7.5 mm to 9.0 mm internal diameter will accommodate most adults. For simplicity, an 8 mm tube can be regarded as the universal adult size. Tubes may be pre-cut or left uncut. Pre-cut tubes save time, but if the entire range is pre-cut, problems may arise with a partially obstructed airway when a smaller diameter tube for that age is required. The average length is 22 cm at the upper incisors for women and 23 cm at the upper incisors for men. In simple terms, the tube length can be estimated as twice the distance from the corner of the mouth to the angle of the jaw. In an adult, the endotracheal tube can remain *in situ* with the cuff inflated for 10–14 days before further intervention such as a tracheostomy is necessary.

In children, the internal diameter is calculated with the formula [age/4 + 4]. For example, a 6-year-old requires a [6/4 + 4] = 5.5 mm tube.

The incidence of vomiting on recovery from anaesthesia is higher in children than adults.

4.10   (A) T (B) T (C) T (D) F (E) F

All victims of significant trauma require oxygen therapy. Most trauma patients have an element of hypoxia or hypovolaemia, or both. Cellular and tissue damage can be minimized by giving supplemental oxygen. Many of the complex biochemical responses in trauma (such as those that result in adult respiratory distress syndrome, or fat embolus syndrome) can be reduced by adequate resuscitation which includes oxygen therapy.

Oxygen should be administered through a tight-fitting Hudson face mask with an attached reservoir bag. This will achieve an inspired concentration of around 85% with a flow rate of 10–15 L/min. Oxygen at 100% can only be delivered through a reservoir-bag-valve-mask or reservoir-bag-valve-tube system, with oxygen at 10–15 L/min.

A full D-sized cylinder set to 15 L/min will last approximately 22 minutes.

4.11   (A) F (B) T (C) T (D) F (E) T

The oropharyngeal airway is sized from the corner of the mouth to the angle of the jaw, and serves to control backwards displacement of the tongue. It provides a free air passage from the lips to the hypopharynx. If the airway is too small it may sit half way down the tongue and aggravate airway obstruction. It is not possible to insert it if the teeth are clenched, and in this situation a nasopharyngeal airway should be inserted.

In adults, the oropharyngeal airway is inserted upside down, then rotated through 180 degrees as it passes over the edge of the hard palate. In children, it must be inserted under direct vision to avoid damage to the soft palate on rotation of the plastic airway. A finger, wooden spatula, or tip of the laryngoscope is used to depress the tongue.

4.12   (A) F (B) F (C) F (D) F (E) T

The nasopharyngeal airway can be a life-saving adjunct, particularly in patients whose airway is compromised and the teeth are clenched. This is often seen in head injuries and epileptics. Care must be taken to introduce it at a right angle to the face, and not be tempted to push it up towards the forehead along the line of the nose. In the latter case, there is a danger of introducing it into the brain through a fractured base of skull. The size is estimated as the one which just introduces the tip of the patient's little finger, or just causes the nostril to blanch.

The end of the device is flanged to prevent it being introduced too far, and this is helped by inserting a safety pin across the top of the device (but not through the nose!).

It is generally not used in children. The reason for this is unclear: there is no specific contraindication, but the airways are not manufactured in paediatric sizes. One can be improvised by cutting down an uncuffed endotracheal tube, using the size 1 mm smaller than the endotracheal requirement for that age.

4.13   (A) F (B) F (C) F (D) F (E) F

The triple airway manoeuvre is a combination of head tilt, chin lift and mouth open. The head tilt is contraindicated in trauma, when a jaw thrust should be done.

Traction applied to the cervical spine could occasionally worsen a cervical cord injury and, for this reason, in-line spinal stabilization is used, and is maintained even after the application of a semi-rigid collar. A head-box, or sandbags + tape, replaces the need for manual immobilization.

Airway management takes priority over cervical spine protection. Occasionally, it is necessary to extend the head in order to open the airway when the jaw thrust is not adequate. If the airway is obstructed, the patient will certainly die, whereas in the majority of cases, you are only immobilizing the cervical spine to protect a suspected rather than a definite injury. The incidence of cervical spine injury is actually about 5% in the unconscious victim of blunt trauma.

An ambulance officer's nightmare is the restless trauma patient who will not cooperate with interventions such as intravenous access, and whose continued movement prevents the adequate stabilization of the cervical spine. Such restlessness may result from hypoxia (airway obstruction; chest injury; head injury), hypovolaemia, inadequate analgesia, or even a full bladder in a patient with a reduced level of response who has received intravenous fluids. It is better to look for the cause of agitation and treat it, than to seek methods of restraint.

4.14 (A) F (B) F (C) F (D) T (E) T

Hypovolaemic shock is divided into four classes. In class III and class IV there is hypotension. Current resuscitation practice (*Advanced Trauma Life Support; Pre-hospital Trauma Life Support*) suggests crystalloid should be used in class I and class II shock, whereas colloid should be the initial fluid of choice in classes III and IV. It should be remembered that blood is needed early in the resuscitation of class III and IV shock. Crystalloid is replaced on a 3:1 basis for blood lost, and colloid is replaced in a 1:1 ratio.

Colloid is a suspension of particles which has an osmotic effect, drawing extravascular fluid into the vascular compartment.

Haemaccel® has a shelf life of approximately 7 years at room temperature. Normal saline is not actually a true 'normal' solution, that is, its salt content is not entirely the same as plasma. It is slightly hypertonic. When given in large volumes it may produce a *hyperchloraemic* (excess chloride: remember, saline is sodium chloride in solution) *acidosis*. The ideal crystalloid to use in resuscitation is Hartman's solution (called Ringer's lactate in the United States).

4.15 (A) T (B) T (C) T (D) F (E) T

The flow through a cannula is governed by four factors:

- The diameter of the cannula
- The length of the cannula
- The viscosity of the fluid
- The pressure applied to the system

These factors are all components of *Poiseuille's law.* The diameter is the most important factor. Flow is proportional to the radius to the power four. This means that if the radius is doubled, the flow rate theoretically increases by 16 times (in practice it does increase, but not by quite this much). Flow is inversely proportional to the length of the cannula, so if the length is doubled the flow is halved. Flow is also inversely proportional to the viscosity (colloids flow more slowly than crystalloids) and to the pressure applied to the system. Infusion rates are also slowed in the cold.

4.16   (A) F (B) F (C) F (D) T (E) T

With an intraosseous infusion fluids are entering a relatively restricted bone marrow compartment, and flow rates by gravity are generally much slower than by the intravenous route. A 50 ml syringe attached to a short connecting tube and a three-way tap are recommended, and fluids and drugs syringed in. It is important not to syringe in too fast under too much pressure as there will be extravasation around the needle. A number of sites can be used including: the anterior surface of the tibia just medial to and below the tibial tuberosity; the lateral aspect of the femoral condyle; just above the medial malleolus; and the lateral aspect of the humeral neck. Generally, the technique is recommended for children up to the age of 6 years, but it has even been used in adults (medial malleolus, or iliac crest).

Should the needle be displaced, an alternate site must be used or further fluid will leak out of the original hole. It is not contraindicated in brittle bone disease, but due caution should be exercised.

The needle is secured by packing dental swabs, for example, between the flange and the skin, and taping the needle in place, then placing the limb in a box splint.

4.17   (A) F (B) F (C) F (D) F (E) T

A laryngeal mask airway can be used in all age groups. A size 1 is suitable for a neonate/infant, and a size 5 in a large adult. One disadvantage is that it will not prevent gastric aspiration, which is why tracheal intubation remains the gold standard. This airway is used extensively in elective anaesthesia (in fact to such an extent that it is now difficult for paramedics to obtain adequate experience of intubation on their hospital attachments), but its role in pre-hospital care is not well developed. It may find a niche for the unconscious patient when there is a lack of equipment or expertise to intubate. It is inserted directly without the use of a laryngoscope. Recent studies have supported its use in hospital cardiac arrest.

The pharyngotracheal lumen airway (PTLA) or Combi-tube, are alternatives to the laryngeal mask.

SHORT ANSWERS

4.18 The causes of airway obstruction include:

- Foreign body (food; broken teeth; dental plate; vomit; blood)
- Tongue (reduced level of response from drugs or head injury; trauma to the lower jaw)
- Mid-face fractures (Le Fort fractures, with posterior displacement of the mid-face)
- Massive facial oedema (burns; anaphylaxis)
- Laryngeal trauma (fractures of the hyoid and thyroid cartilages)
- Infection (epiglottitis; quinsy – tonsillar abscess)
- Blocked artificial airway (endotracheal tube; tracheostomy tube)

4.19 The options are:

- Bag-valve-mask system
- Laryngeal mask airway
- Pharyngotracheal lumen airway (PTLA)/Combi-tube
- Needle or surgical cricothyrotomy

When intubation is difficult or impractical, and the transport time to hospital is short, bag-valve-mask ventilation is appropriate, together with rapid transport. An oropharyngeal or nasopharyngeal airway will be a useful adjunct.

The laryngeal mask airway is discussed in question 4.17. The Combi-tube is a double-lumen tube passed blindly through the mouth. Ventilation is possible whether the tube enters the trachea or the oesophagus. The PTLA is a similar device: the longer tube is designed to enter the oesophagus and is cuffed, but should it enter the trachea, ventilation can then take place via a cuffed endotracheal tube.

A cricothyrotomy is indicated when there is a life-threatening airway obstruction and both positional manoeuvres and intubation have failed. It is, therefore, a 'technique of failure'. In the pre-hospital setting, it would first be appropriate to attempt a needle cricothyrotomy, and only proceed to a surgical cricothyrotomy if rapid transport to hospital cannot be achieved.

Current paramedic practice in the United Kingdom allows bag-valve-mask ventilation or intubation. It is likely that needle cricothyrotomy and the laryngeal mask airway will be added to this armamentarium in the future.

4.20 The first priority, as always, is *safety*: yourself, the scene and the casualty. In the primary survey, the airway is opened by jaw thrust: head tilt is not used here as there is a risk of cervical spine injury. Associated injuries in general are common in burns as people will jump out of a window to escape the flames, or may stumble and fall downstairs in the smoke. This patient requires assisted ventilation with high-flow oxygen, although once removed from the toxic environment, respirations may recover spontaneously. Intubation could only be attempted if the patient has no airway reflexes.

Once airway and breathing have been controlled, the circulation and disability are assessed. Urgent transfer to hospital is required. There is a risk of airway obstruction owing to oedema from the inhalation of hot gases, and elective intubation in hospital when there are signs of upper airway burn is a better course of action than a surgical airway once the obstruction has occurred.

Monitoring on the way to hospital should include ECG, and respiratory rate. Pulse oximetry may be unreliable if there is associated carbon monoxide poisoning.

PICTURE QUIZ

4.21 Needle cricothyrotomy is an airway technique to overcome upper airway obstruction unrelieved by manual manoeuvres, and where endotracheal intubation is not possible. Access is via the cricothyroid membrane with a large bore (14g) cannula on a syringe. As the cannula is advanced, the syringe is aspirated continuously until there is a free flow of air. On its own the needle is *not* an adequate airway, and oxygen must be jetted in from a cylinder at 15 L/min. The connection to the cannula can be achieved with a 'Y-connector', a three-way tap, or tapered oxygen tubing forced into the barrel of a 2 ml syringe and a hole cut in the side of the tubing. Whatever delivery system is chosen, it is wise to prepare it in advance. This is a ventilation technique and the chest should be seen to rise when oxygen is jetted in for 1 second: the chest is then allowed to recoil for 4 seconds.

PHARMACOLOGY AND POISONING

Refer to Chapters 8 and 16 of
Emergency Care: A Textbook for Paramedics.

MULTIPLE CHOICE

5.1   The following are true:

A.   Pharmacokinetics is the study of the effects of drugs on the body

B.   The Home Office is responsible for licensing drugs

C.   The use of prescription only medicines (POM) is controlled by the Medicines Act of 1968

D.   Metaclopramide is a generic name

E.   Opiates may only be administered by a doctor

5.2   The following drugs are correctly matched with their side effects:

A.   Lignocaine   Seizures

B.   Aspirin   Bronchospasm

C.   Naloxone   Coma

D.   Glyceryl trinitrate   Headache

E.   Nalbuphine   Hypotension

5.3   The effects of adrenaline include:

A.   Tachycardia

B.   Bronchoconstriction

C.   Hypertension

D.   Increased coronary perfusion

E.   Anxiety

5.4   Aspirin:

A.   Is predominantly metabolized by the kidney

B.   Is antipyretic

C.   Is contraindicated in patients with chronic obstructive pulmonary disease

D.   Causes ringing or whistling in the ears (tinnitus)

E.   Is contraindicated in children <12 years

5.5   Atropine:

A.   May precipitate urinary retention

B.   Is effective enterally

C.   Is given in 1 mg aliquots in asystole

D.   Causes blurred vision

E.   Is a cholinergic drug

5.6   Indications for adrenaline include:

A.   Asystole

B.   Asthma

C.   Neurogenic shock

D.   Hypovolaemic shock

E.   Self-administration in anaphylaxis

5.7   Entonox is an appropriate analgesic for:

A.   A 56-year-old with a myocardial infarction

B.   A motorcyclist with crush injuries to the chest

C.   A woman in labour

D.   A SCUBA diver with a Colles' fracture

E.   Use by mountain rescue teams

5.8   Oxytocin:

A.   Relaxes the uterus

B.   May be given by SC, IM or IV injections

C.   Stimulates lactation

D.   May cause abdominal pain and vomiting

E.   Is a naturally occurring hormone

5.9   Glucagon:

A.   Causes bradycardia

B.   Is usually given IV

C.   Reverses the effects of β-agonists, such as salbutamol

D.   Is effective in all patients with hypoglycaemia

E.   Is contraindicated in asthma

5.10   Lignocaine:

A.   Causes vomiting and drowsiness

B.   Is the drug of first choice in ventricular tachycardia

C.   Reduces the fibrillation threshold

D.   Is metabolized in the liver

E.   Increases the likelihood of successful cardioversion from ventricular fibrillation

5.11   Nalbuphine:

A.   Is a pure opiate antagonist

B.   Is not associated with respiratory depression

C.   Is contraindicated in opiate dependency

D.   Does not cause nausea and vomiting

E.   Cannot be given after Entonox

5.12 Nitrous oxide:

A. Is marketed as Entonox

B. Causes central nervous system depression

C. Is contraindicated in gastrointestinal obstruction

D. Is eliminated unchanged through the lungs

E. Must not be used in asthmatics

5.13 Ipecacuanha:

A. May cause prolonged vomiting

B. Is contraindicated for home use

C. May produce drowsiness

D. Is indicated in benzodiazepine overdose

E. Is associated with aspiration pneumonitis

5.14 Concerning benzodiazepine overdose:

A. Naloxone is the specific antagonist

B. Treatment may precipitate seizures

C. Intravenous overdose is recognized

D. Prolonged duration of action is a problem

E. It is made worse by concomitant alcohol

5.15 Effects of tricyclic antidepressant poisoning include:

A. *Torsades de pointes*

B. Metabolic alkalosis

C. Coma

D. Hypotension

E. Dilated pupils

5.16 You are called to a patient aged 24 who is unconscious. He is wearing a *Medic-Alert*® bracelet which informs you he is a diabetic. Place the following priorities in the order in which you would perform them:

1. A blood sugar estimation

2. Obtaining background information

3. Establishing a patent airway

4. Rapid evacuation to hospital

5. Establishing an intravenous line

A. 1–4–5–2–3

B. 5–2–4–1–3

C. 3–5–1–2–4

D. 3–4–2–5–1

E. 3–2–4–1–5

5.17 The following are true regarding drug overdose:

A. Naloxone has a longer duration of action than morphine

B. Dilated pupils are a useful diagnostic feature

C. Patients may be treated against their will

D. Hypotension may occur

E. Patients must be reported to the police for possessing a controlled drug

SHORT ANSWERS

5.18 List the different routes of administration of drugs, and give for each route any relevant advantages or disadvantages.

5.19 Define the folowing terms:

- Distribution
- Bioavailability
- Elimination (clearance)

5.20 Write short notes on *Laburnum* poisoning.

5.21 You are called to a road traffic accident involving a man on a motorbike who has a closed fracture of the shaft of femur. Discuss the different methods of pain control available to you with their advantages and disadvantages.

5.22 For each of the following effects give one drug which will produce the given problem in overdose:

- Tachycardia
- Decreased respiratory rate
- Hypotension
- Increased respiratory rate
- Pupillary dilatation

PICTURE QUIZ

5.23   What are the differences between these two systems?

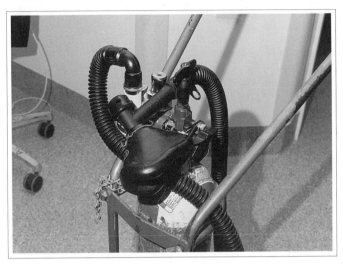

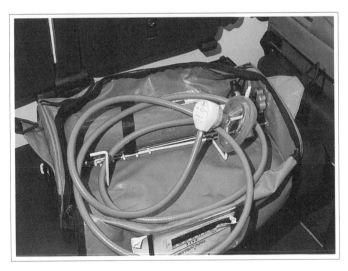

5.24 A small child has swallowed one of these. What would you do?

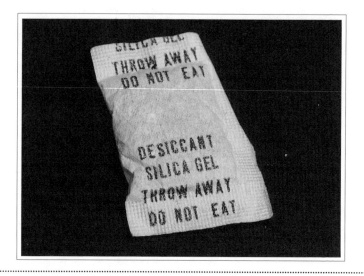

CASE HISTORY

5.25 You are called to a bedsit in an area of the city popular with students. A tearful girl shows you into a bedroom where a second girl is lying unconscious on the bed.

1. What is your differential diagnosis?

2. How would you reach a definite diagnosis?

3. What are the initial management priorities?

PHARMACOLOGY AND POISONING

MULTIPLE CHOICE

5.1 (A) F (B) F (C) T (D) T (E) F

Pharmacodynamics is the study of the biochemical and physiological effects of a drug on the body; *pharmocokinetics* is the study of how a drug gets into, around and out of the body ('the effects of the body on a drug'). The authority responsible for licensing drugs in the UK is the Department of Health. Metaclopramide is a *generic* name: 'Maxalon' and 'Primperan' are its *trade* names, and its *chemical* name is *4 amino-5 chloro-N-[2 diethylamino]ethyl-1,2 methoxybenzamine.* Opiates (drugs derived from opium) such as morphine are usually administered by doctors, but a concession exists in the UK for these drugs to be carried and administered by first-aid-trained members of a mountain rescue team. Outside the UK, morphine is administered by ambulance personnel (e.g. Australia). Nalbuphine is a synthetic morphine-like drug, and is used by ambulance services in the UK.

5.2 (A) T (B) T (C) F (D) T (E) T

Naloxone is a specific opiate antagonist used to reverse the effect of morphine, diamorphine (heroin), and other related drugs, such as nalbuphine (note: nalbuphine is only partially reversed by naloxone). Like morphine, nalbuphine may produce hypotension. Aspirin should be avoided in asthmatics as a small proportion are aspirin sensitive and an asthmatic attack will be precipitated. GTN tablets or spray commonly cause headache secondary to cerebral vasodilation: this should resolve rapidly on spitting out the tablet.

5.3   (A) T (B) F (C) T (D) T (E) F

Adrenaline is a sympathomimetic drug (reproduces the effects of the activated sympathetic nervous system) whose most important effects in resuscitation are to increase both coronary and cerebral perfusion. Adrenaline causes bronchodilation, and has been used in the treatment of life-threatening asthma.

5.4   (A) F (B) T (C) F (D) T (E) T

Aspirin is metabolized in the blood and liver, and is excreted by the kidneys. Like paracetamol it is antipyretic (reduces temperature in fever), but it is contraindicated in children as it has been asociated with the development of Reye's syndrome (a potentially fatal liver and brain disease). Aspirin is also relatively contraindicated in asthma, as it may precipitate bronchospasm (see question 5.2). Tinnitus is a well-described feature of aspirin overdose.

5.5   (A) T (B) F (C) F (D) T (E) F

Atropine is an anticholinergic drug, whose side effects include pupil dilation and blurred vision, dry mouth, retention of urine and confusion. It must be given parenterally. The dose in asystole is 3 mg once only.

5.6   (A) T (B) F (C) F (D) F (E) T

Adrenaline has been used in the treatment of life-threatening asthma, but it is not recommended for routine pre-hospital use. The treatment of neurogenic shock includes cautious intravenous fluids, and atropine. Atopic ('allergic', often referring to the coexistence of asthma, eczema and hayfever) patients who react badly to a common allergen (allergy-producing substance, e.g. animal fur, wasp sting) may carry adrenaline for self-administered subcutaneous injection.

5.7   (A) T (B) F (C) T (D) F (E) F

Entonox (a 50:50 mixture of oxygen and nitrous oxide) is contraindicated in patients at risk of decompression sickness (also known as 'the bends', or Caisson disease), and in patients with a chest injury (even a small pneumothorax may rapidly tension and threaten life). Entonox is not appropriate for use by mountain rescue teams, because of the logistical problem of carrying heavy cylinders.

5.8   (A) F (B) T (C) T (D) T (E) T

Oxytocin causes rapid uterine contraction and stimulates lactation. It is marketed in combination with ergometrine which has a more sustained effect on the uterus (oxytocin + ergometrine = Syntometrine). It is used routinely for the third stage of labour, or as an emergency treatment for post-partum haemorrhage. Syntometrine may be administered by paramedics with obstetric modular training.

5.9   (A) F (B) F (C) F (D) F (E) F

Glucagon is a naturally occurring hormone which breaks down glycogen stores liberating glucose, and stimulates the heart increasing the rate and contractility. It is not contraindicated in asthma, and is used in the treatment of β-blocker (e.g. atenolol, propanolol) overdose. Glucagon may not be effective in alcohol-induced hypoglycaemia, as alcoholics characteristically have low or absent glycogen stores.

5.10   (A) T (B) T (C) F (D) T (E) F

Side effects of lignocaine include perioral tingling, nausea, vomiting, bradycardia, hypotension and seizures. Lignocaine is the drug of choice in patients who have VT with a pulse (for pulseless VT follow the VF protocol). One mechanism of action is to raise the fibrillation threshold by stabilizing cell membranes. For this reason, it is now believed that lignocaine *reduces* the likelihood of successful cardioversion from VF.

5.11   (A) F (B) F (C) T (D) F (E) F

Nalbuphine is a synthetic opioid which may cause nausea, vomiting, hypotension and respiratory depression. As it is not a controlled drug, it has an attraction for use in pre-hospital care. However, this must be tempered against the fact that it is not as effective as morphine, and since it is a 'partial antagonist' it will reduce the effect of morphine given later by a doctor (as it will compete with the morphine receptors). Additionally, it cannot be completely reversed by naloxone.

5.12   (A) T (B) T (C) T (D) T (E) F

Nitrous oxide does cause CNS depression, but this is not a problem when it is self-administered. The gas is eliminated unchanged through the lungs and, although it is not contraindicated in asthmatics, it should not be given to any patient who requires high-flow oxygen.

5.13 (A) T (B) T (C) T (D) F (E) T

15% of children who receive ipecacuanha will develop prolonged vomiting, diarrhoea and drowsiness resulting in a risk of aspiration and pneumonitis.

5.14 (A) F (B) T (C) T (D) T (E) T

Naloxone (Narcan®) is a specific opiate antagonist. Intravenous abuse of benzodiazepines has recently led to the removal from prescription of gel containing temazepam preparations ('wobbly eggs'). The duration of action of some benzodiazepines may be prolonged and the effects of overdose will be exacerbated by concomitant alcohol consumption.

5.15 (A) T (B) F (C) T (D) T (E) T

Overdose of tricyclic antidepressants is relatively common, and is associated with a wide range of tachydysrhythmias (abnormal and fast heart rhythms) including *Torsades de pointes*. A metabolic acidosis, hypotension, dilated pupils and coma are all common features of severe overdose.

5.16 3–5–1–2–4 = C

5.17 (A) F (B) T (C) F (D) T (E) F

Naloxone has a much shorter half-life than most opiates, as a consequence of which the signs of opiate poisoning may recur some time after treatment as the antidote 'wears off'. This may be a problem with patients who awaken aggressive and uncooperative, refuse further treatment, only to collapse again later. Hypotension may occur and pinpoint pupils are a useful diagnostic sign in opiate overdose. Dilated pupils may be a diagnostic indicator of tricyclic antidepressant overdose. Patients may not be treated against their will (unless a police or hospital order is in force whereby the patient is treated involuntarily under the Mental Health Act), and to inform the police that a patient is in possession of an illegal drug would be a breach of confidentiality.

SHORT ANSWERS

5.18   The different routes of drug administration are:

1. Enteral (via the alimentary tract)

   - *Oral.* Convenient and easy to administer, but may have slow absorption. Contra-indicated when the patient is still to be assessed for urgent surgery. An example pre-hospital is aspirin 300 mg chewed after a suspected myocardial infarction.
   - *Rectal.* Useful when the patient is unresponsive, nauseated or unable to swallow. An example is diazepam 5–10 mg administered for convulsions.
   - *Sublingual.* Rapid absorption and onset of action. An example is GTN tablets or spray used for an angina attack.
   - *Buccal.* Again, rapid absorption and onset of action. An alternative to the sub-lingual route for administering nitrates. Here a tablet is pressed against the upper gum and becomes adherent. Such tablets are not currently available for use by the ambulance service.

2. Parenteral (non-alimentary route)

   - *Dermal.* Some drugs can be released slowly through a skin patch. These include hormone replacements and nitrates. A nitrate patch on the chest *must* be removed before defibrillation to prevent a risk of explosion.
   - *Subcutaneous.* This route is used for injecting insulin in diabetes, and is an alternative to intramuscular injection for adrenaline in anaphylaxis. Absorption is relatively slow (particularly in shock, when the skin perfusion is poor), and it is a useful route for drugs that may have a rapid and profound effect when absorbed too quickly.
   - *Intramuscular.* This is a simple route, with few complications when the upper outer quadrant of the buttock is used. Absorption is faster than subcutaneous injection, but is still unreliable in shock: opiate analgesia (nalbuphine, morphine) is best given intravenously because of this erratic absorption, either following trauma or a myocardial infarct. Glucagon is given by this route in hypoglycaemia, and adrenaline can be given intramuscularly in anaphylaxis.
   - *Intravenous.* This route is used when an immediate response to administered drugs is required, for example, in cardiac arrest.
   - *Intraosseous.* This is a very useful alternative to the intravenous route in children (< 6 years), if intravenous access proves difficult.
   - *Endotracheal.* In cardiac arrest, adrenaline and atropine may be given down the endotracheal route in 2–3 times the intravenous dose. It is less effective than the intravenous route.
   - *Nebulizer.* This delivers a high concentration of drug to its specific place of action. It is a valuable method of delivering bronchodilators in acute asthma.
   - *Intracardiac.* This was a method for delivering drugs in cardiac arrest, via a long needle under the xiphisternum. *It is no longer recommended.*

5.19 The *distribution* of a drug is the way it is divided between different body tisues.

The *bioavailability* is the amount of that drug available to carry out its intended pharmacological action, after the body has acted upon it (and perhaps altered its structure).

Elimination (or *clearance*) is the way the drug is removed from the body, for example, via the kidneys, liver, lungs or faeces.

5.20 *Laburnum* poisoning is common in the UK. If more than ten seeds are ingested, the following symptoms may develop:

- Burning in the mouth and throat
- Nausea and vomiting
- Abdominal pain
- Diarrhoea
- Drowsiness and delirium
- Incoordination
- Twitching
- Coma

Fatalities are extremely rare. Pre-hospital treatment is directed simply towards the support of 'ABC'.

With ingestion of a plant, or fungus, it is always helpful to take a sample to the hospital to assist in identification.

5.21 Available methods of analgesia include:

1. *Reassurance.* The appearance of the emergency services will provide reassurance to the casualty, and verbal reasurance should be continued throughout the rescue.

2. *Splintage.* This patient has a fractured femur. A traction splint will not only reduce pain, but it will reduce blood loss (by up to 30%), and minimize secondary neurovascular damage. A traction splint should not be used if an unstable pelvic fracture is also suspected. In services where traction splints are not used, or when a 'scoop and run' is required because of more pressing airway, breathing or circulation problems, a simple long box splint may be used, or even just splintage to the uninjured leg with triangular bandages.

3. *Entonox.* This is a strong analgesic, equivalent to 10 mg morphine. It has particular use in facilitating extrication, or to assist in the gentle manipulation of the limb during splintage. The temptation can be to assume that it is working after only a few breaths, whereas it takes several minutes before its maximal effect is achieved. It is contra-indicated if the patient requires high-flow oxygen, if the patient is unable to cooperate, or if there is a chest injury (a pneumothorax may tension).

4. *Intravenous agents.* Morphine is not currently available for use by ambulance personnel in the UK, although it is used by other services world-wide (for example, Australia). The alternative is a weaker, synthetic morphine-like drug called nalbuphine. This can still cause respiratory depression, but it is not fully reversed by naloxone.

5.22 The table below links common side effects of drugs taken in overdose:

Problem in overdose	Example drugs
Tachycardia	Tricyclic antidepressants, amphetamines, LSD, Ecstasy
Bradycardia	Beta-blockers
Hypotension	Tricyclic antidepressants, opiates, beta-blockers
Decreased respiratory rate	Opiates (morphine, heroin, codeine)
Increased respiratory rate	Aspirin
Pupillary dilatation	Tricyclic antidepressants

PICTURE QUIZ

5.23 Entonox is the original delivery system for a 50:50 mixture of nitrous oxide and oxygen. The demand valve is located at the cylinder, so a significant negative pressure must be generated by the patient to trigger the system. With Nitronox the demand valve is located at the mask, so it is easier for the patient to trigger.

5.24 Silica gel is non-toxic and is commonly found in electrical or optical instrument packaging as an absorbent. Lists exist of non-toxic household substances that are commonly ingested, but if such a list was not available the ambulance crew would have no option but to seek medical advice at hospital. No treatment other than reassurance is appropriate in this case.

CASE HISTORY

5.25 The differential diagnosis (common causes in this age group) is:

- Hypoglycaemia
- Epilepsy (post-ictal)
- Drug overdose
    Opiates (e.g. morphine, heroin)
    Antidepressants
    Benzodiazepines (sleeping tablets, e.g. temazepam)

Hypoglycaemia would be strongly suggested by a bracelet that says 'DIABETIC'. It should be excluded by a finger-prick blood glucose test. The best clue to epilepsy is in the history. Did someone witness the clonic movements of a fit? Has the patient been incontinent or bitten their tongue? A warning bracelet may also be worn by an epileptic. Drug overdose would be suspected if there are empty pill bottles or blister packs, or syringe and needle, or a suicide note. Did the patient intend to be found? If not (doors locked), this means that there was strong motivation for suicide, rather than just a 'cry for help'.

Further clues may be present on examination, for example, constricted pupils (opiates) or dilated pupils (tricyclic antidepressants).

Whatever the cause of the collapse, the priorities are the same, namely *Safety–ABC*. Once these priorities have been followed, attention can be turned to the specific cause of collapse, and treatment given pre-hospital where appropriate (naloxone for opiate abuse; glucagon or glucose for hypoglycaemia).

MEDICAL EMERGENCIES

Refer to Chapters 9, 14 and 15 of
Emergency Care: A Textbook for Paramedics.

MULTIPLE CHOICE

6.1 **Obstruction of the smaller airways in asthma is a combined result of:**

A. Mucosal oedema

B. Mucus plugging

C. Hyperinflated chest

D. Bronchiolar smooth muscle constriction

E. Lung bullae

6.2 **The following are normal respiratory values in a healthy adult male at rest:**

A. Tidal volume of 1000 ml

B. Minute volume of 5000 ml

C. Anatomical dead space of 150 ml

D. An oxygen saturation of 93% on air at sea level

E. Peak expiratory flow rate of 200 L/min

6.3 **Signs that indicate an acute asthmatic attack in a 14-year-old boy is *not* life-threatening include:**

A. A pulse of 130 per minute

B. Central cyanosis

C. A noticeable reduction in the radial pulse on inspiration

D. A chest without wheeze

E. A respiratory rate of 12 per minute

6.4 **The treatment of anaphylaxis resulting from a bee sting may include:**

A. A needle cricothyrotomy

B. The administration of intramuscular adrenaline

C. The administration of intravenous adrenaline

D. Removal of the bee sting and sucking the venom from the wound

E. A salbutamol nebulizer

6.5 **With regard to meningococcal septicaemia:**

A. This condition tends to develop insidiously over 2–3 days

B. The associated rash is characteristically urticarial

C. Penicillin needs to be given as soon as the diagnosis is made

D. The ambulance crew transporting the patient must receive prophylactic antibiotics

E. Paramedic staff can be effectively vaccinated against this disease

6.6 **The following are features of a subarachnoid haemorrhage:**

A. Sudden onset of a severe headache, like a blow to the head

B. Neck stiffness

C. Photophobia

D. It is often a result of a ruptured intracranial aneurysm

E. Prognosis for recovery is generally good

6.7 **The following are true of diabetic hypoglycaemia:**

A. It may be caused by an overdose of insulin

B. Hypoglycaemic coma is less common than hyperglycaemic coma

C. Small children respond poorly to glucagon

D. The first sign may be aggressiveness

E. There is an associated bradycardia

SHORT ANSWERS

6.8 List the clinical signs of acute appendicitis.

6.9 Write short notes on the treatment of severe asthma.

6.10 Make a table of the differences between left ventricular failure (LVF) and chronic obstructive pulmonary disease (COPD).

PICTURE QUIZ

6.11 This is a home nebulizer. What is the difference between it and the system you would use, and which system is better?

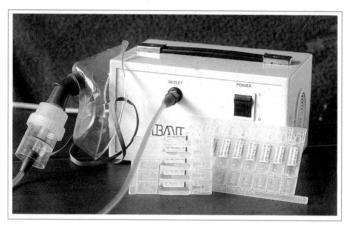

6.12 What is this drug used for? What initial dose would you use in (a) a 2-year-old, (b) a 6-year-old, (c) an adult?

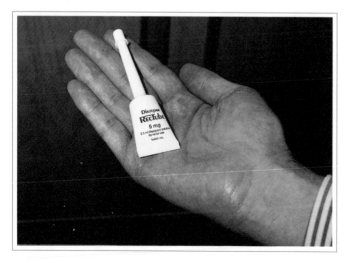

CASE HISTORY

You are working a night shift with a partner from another station who is providing cover for leave. You are called to the home of a 24-year-old woman with severe lower right-sided abdominal pain. When you arrive you find her writhing in agony on the lounge floor. She says she has had two operations on the abdomen in the last year, one for suspected appendicitis, and one for a suspected twisted ovarian cyst. When you gently touch her abdomen you feel that the muscles are tense and she shouts out in pain.

1. What are your actions?
2. What are the possible diagnoses?

Your partner takes you to one side and says that he recognizes this woman and is sure that he has treated her in another area for the same condition. What diagnosis might you consider now?

MEDICAL EMERGENCIES

MULTIPLE CHOICE

6.1 **(A) T (B) T (C) F (D) T (E) F**

Oedema, mucus plugging and bronchial smooth muscle constriction are the principal causes of lower airway obstruction in asthma. Treatment is directed towards reducing these:

Constriction	Smooth muscle relaxants, e.g. salbutamol
Oedema	Anti-inflammatory agents, e.g. steroids
Mucus plugging	Rehydration and physiotherapy

6.2 **(A) F (B) T (C) T (D) F (E) F**

The normal tidal volume is about 400 ml. Oxygen saturation at sea level should be 97–100% in healthy lungs. The normal adult male peak flow rate is about 600 L/min.

6.3 **(A) F (B) F (C) F (D) F (E) F**

A decrease in the radial pulse on inspiration is known as *pulsus paradoxus*. It occurs in severe asthma or cardiac tamponade. A silent chest is ominous, and implies insufficient air is moving to produce a wheeze. An asthmatic with a normal respiratory rate is tiring and requires ventilatory support.

6.4 **(A) T (B) T (C) T (D) F (E) T**

Following anaphylaxis the upper airway may swell and obstruct, necessitating a cricothyrotomy. Adrenaline is usually administered by deep intramuscular injection, but it may be given intravenously in a severe crisis (but it must be given slowly, and in the diluted 1:10,000 solution). Symptoms and signs of bronchoconstriction, such as shortness of breath with wheeze, are treated the same as asthma.

6.5 **(A) F (B) F (C) T (D) F (E) F**

Meningococcal disease (which includes *meningococcal meningitis* and *meningococcal septicaemia*) characteristically develops rapidly, over a number of hours. The rash of meningococcal septicaemia is purpuric (bleeding under the skin which does not blanch on pressure), and is often widespread. The ambulance attendant does not require antibiotics unless mouth-to-mouth ventilation has been provided. Vaccination is only effective against two of the three strains of the meningococcus (strains A and C), and unfortunately most cases in the UK are from strain B (although strain C is becoming increasingly important).

6.6 **(A) T (B) T (C) T (D) T (E) F**

In a subarachnoid haemorrhage there is bleeding outside the brain between the layers of the enveloping meninges. Irritation of the meninges by blood causes 'meningism', which manifests as photophobia and neck stiffness. Headache is usually severe and of sudden onset. A common cause of a subarachnoid haemorrhage is the rupture of a developmental aneurysm (dilated blood vessel) located in the circular arterial network at the base of the brain (rupture of a Berry aneurysm in the Circle of Willis).

6.7 **(A) T (B) F (C) T (D) T (E) F**

Hypoglycaemia in a diabetic may be the result of excessive insulin, inadequate food or excessive exertion. Children respond poorly to glucagon, which mobilizes the liver stores of glycogen and converts them into glucose, because glycogen stores are often low. In childhood illness, hypoglycaemia is common, irrespective of the cause of the illness, because in a stressed body the glycogen stores are rapidly utilized. The associated features of hypoglycaemia are tachycardia, pallor, sweating, and aggression or irritability developing into a progressive loss of consciousness.

SHORT ANSWERS

6.8 The features of acute appendicitis are:

- Central abdominal pain, shifting after several hours to the right iliac fossa (lower right side of the abdomen)
- Tenderness in the same distribution with muscular guarding (muscles tighten on pressing) and rebound tenderness (worsening of pain on suddenly removing hand from abdomen)
- Loss of appetite
- Fever
- Change of bowel habit (constipation or diarrhoea)
- Tachycardia

6.9 The treatment of severe asthma pre-hospital is:

- Reassure
- Sit up if conscious (almost certainly will already be sitting up)
- High-flow oxygen
- Nebulized β_2-agonist (salbutamol or terbutaline)
- Support airway and ventilation if required

Remember: asthmatics die of hypoxia. ALWAYS give oxygen.

6.10 The differences between acute left ventricular failure and an acute exacerbation of chronic obstructive pulmonary disease are given in the table below:

Acute LVF	Exacerbation COPD
History	
History of ischaemic heart disease $\pm$ waking at night short of breath, relieved by sitting up $\pm$ shortness of breath on exertion (stairs)	Known chronic bronchitic
Associated features	
• Chest pain • Dysrhythmia • Hypotension • Pink, frothy sputum	• Fever (if precipitating infection) • Cough productive of green/yellow sputum
Examination	
• Widespread inspiratory crackles • Wheeze less prominent	• Hyperinflated chest • Breathing with pursed lips • Wheeze prominent

PICTURE QUIZ

6.11 Home nebulizers are often driven by air. Nebulizers used by the ambulance service and in hospital are driven by oxygen. Asthmatics die from hypoxia. A nebulizer used in the emergency treatment of asthma should always be driven by oxygen, not air.

6.12 Rectal diazepam is used pre-hospital for the treatment of convulsions. It is a convenient route to deliver a drug when intravenous access is difficult, for example, in the fitting patient. The dose is 5 mg rectally in children 1–3 years, and 10 mg in older children and adults (5 mg in the elderly).

CASE HISTORY

Your actions would include:

- Obtain a medical history
- Establish baseline observations
- Provide reassurance
- Consider analgesia (e.g. nalbuphine)
- Transport to hospital

The diagnoses you would consider are:

- Appendicitis, but the appendix has been removed
- Twisted ovarian cyst, which could be recurrent
- Inflammatory bowel disease (Crohn's disease), which is by nature relapsing
- Pelvic inflammatory disease (infection of pelvic organs, often *Chlamydia*)
- Munchausen's syndrome. This is where the patient invents symptoms, which are often surgical in nature, and which may result in fruitless operations. You would have no confirmation that the patient truly had appendicitis or an ovarian cyst, so it is worth considering this diagnosis, but it is a diagnosis of exclusion: *rule other things out first.*

With the further history of possible frequent hospital attendances with painful abdominal conditions, you should consider if this patient is using fictitious symptoms in order to receive opiate analgesics. Such patients often attend a number of hospitals to reduce the chance of detection, the so-called 'hospital hopper'.

CARDIAC EMERGENCIES

Refer to Chapters 10, 11, 12 and 13 of
Emergency Care: A Textbook for Paramedics.

MULTIPLE CHOICE

7.1   Regarding the heart:

A.   The blood supply to the SA node is from the right coronary artery

B.   The left ventricle is predominantly supplied by the left coronary artery

C.   The cardiac veins run off the coronary sinus

D.   The coronary arteries run from the left atrium

E.   The pulmonary vein carries deoxygenated blood back to the heart

7.2   In an adult:

A.   A single cardiac cycle lasts about 800 milliseconds

B.   The circulating blood volume is 8 litres

C.   The ventricular stroke volume is 70–80 ml at rest

D.   Cardiac output is 10 L/min at rest

E.   Tachycardia is defined as a heart rate greater than 100 per minute

7.3   Concerning the ECG:

A.   AVR is the right leg lead

B.   The standard leads are II, III and aVF

C.   Lead AVR is always negative

D.   Lead III is most appropriate for pre-hospital cardiac monitoring

E.   The normal paper speed is 50 mm/s

7.4 Pulse oximetry:

A. Is a reliable guide to the severity of carbon monoxide poisoning

B. Is not reliable in patients with dark skin

C. Is unaffected by the presence of nail varnish

D. May be used to monitor the reduction of a displaced limb fracture

E. Is unaffected by temperature

7.5 Regarding pulse oximetry:

A. Normal oxygen saturation is >97% on air

B. Oxygen saturation is lower in smokers

C. Alveolar hypoventilation may be monitored

D. Readings are affected by bright light

E. The progress of respiratory failure may be monitored

7.6 Concerning defibrillator batteries:

A. Lead–acid batteries hold their charge for prolonged periods

B. Nickel–cadmium cells lose charge rapidly if unused

C. Lead–acid batteries must be fully discharged before recharging

D. Nickel–cadmium cells require regular conditioning

E. Dry batteries are used on first responder defibrillators

7.7 Concerning cardiac arrest in adults:

A. It is usually secondary to a metabolic disturbance

B. Asystole is the commonest primary dysrhythmia

C. Pre-hospital the first priority is clearing the *airway*

D. A precordial thump should always be given

E. It may result from opiate overdose

7.8   Precordial thump:

A.   Is indicated in electromechanical dissociation (EMD)

B.   Delivers about 100 J of energy

C.   Is performed over the sternum

D.   May be used to 'pace' an asystolic patient

E.   May convert ventricular fibrillation (VF) into asystole

7.9   Asystole:

A.   Has a survival rate approaching 20%

B.   Should be paced when there is P-wave activity

C.   Is treated with atropine 1 mg every cycle of the arrest protocol

D.   May respond to a precordial thump

E.   May revert to sinus rhythm on coughing

7.10   Causes of electromechanical dissociation include:

A.   Tension pneumothorax

B.   β-blocker overdose

C.   Hypothermia

D.   Pulmonary embolism

E.   Hypocalcaemia

7.11   Sodium bicarbonate:

A.   May exacerbate intracellular acidosis

B.   Increases tissue oxygen availability

C.   May produce tissue necrosis if infused extravascularly

D.   Is indicated in prolonged pre-hospital cardiac arrest

E.   Should not be given through the same line as calcium gluconate

7.12   Risk factors for ischaemic heart disease include:

A.   Stress

B.   Hypertension

C.   Familial hypercholesterolaemia

D.   Diabetes mellitus

E.   Obesity

7.13   Immediately following myocardial infarction, the ECG:

A.   May show T wave inversion

B.   May be normal

C.   Will show ST segment depression in the corresponding leads

D.   May demonstrate complete heart block

E.   Will show Q waves

7.14   Symptoms of myocardial infarction include:

A.   Vomiting

B.   Headache

C.   Sweating

D.   Faintness

E.   Palpitation

7.15   Concerning drugs in myocardial infarction:

A.   Metaclopramide is the antiemetic of choice

B.   Aspirin should be given routinely unless contraindicated

C.   Cyclizine may cause coronary vasoconstriction

D.   The dose of atropine for bradycardia is 3 mg

E.   Prochlorperazine may cause severe hypotension when given intravenously

7.16   **With regard to pre-hospital thrombolysis:**

A.   The mortality of myocardial infarction may be reduced

B.   Effectiveness is increased when combined with aspirin

C.   Anistreplase is the drug of choice

D.   A past history of peptic ulceration is an absolute contraindication

E.   Ventricular tachycardia may occur during myocardial reperfusion

7.17   **Features of dissecting aortic aneurysm include:**

A.   A past history of hypertension

B.   Pain similar to myocardial infarction

C.   Haematuria

D.   Paraplegia

E.   ECG signs of myocardial infarction

7.18   **Causes of cardiac tamponade include:**

A.   Trauma

B.   Myocardial infarction

C.   Tuberculosis

D.   Carcinoma of the bronchus

E.   Following thoracic surgery

7.19   **The following diagnoses are correctly matched with their treatment:**

A.   Complete heart block   Atropine

B.   Ventricular fibrillation   DC shock

C.   Junctional tachycardia   Lignocaine

D.   Second-degree heart block   Adenosine

E.   Ventricular tachycardia (with pulse)   Synchronized DC shock

7.20 **The following manoeuvres will cause the heart to slow:**

A.   Pressure on the eyeball

B.   Carotid sinus massage

C.   Heimlich manoeuvre

D.   Valsalva manoeuvre

E.   Bag of ice on the face

SHORT ANSWERS

7.21 **Draw the cardiac action potential and describe its components.**

7.22 **Draw a diagram of the cardiac conducting system.**

7.23 **Write short notes on the presentation and initial management of pulmonary embolism.**

PICTURE QUIZ

7.24 **Label the ECG complex below and indicate the significance of each component.**

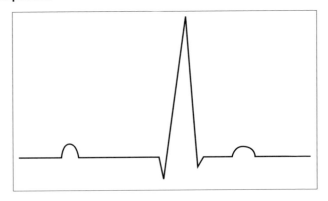

7.25a–d Identify these rhythms.

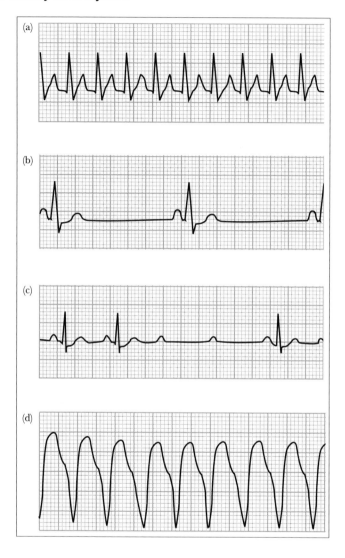

7.26 You apply a cardiac monitor to a patient in cardiac arrest. The screen is as shown. What do you do?

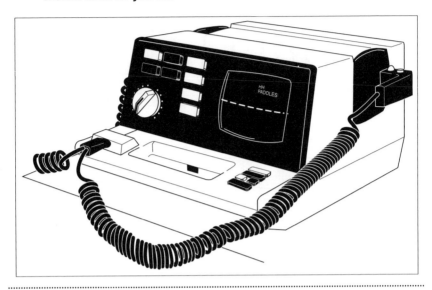

CASE HISTORY

Following an emergency call, you arrive in the car park of a riverside pub. A young male has been pulled from the water. He is very cold and your defibrillator monitor shows VF. Discuss the problems involved in managing this patient.

CARDIAC EMERGENCIES

MULTIPLE CHOICE

7.1 **(A) T (B) T (C) F (D) F (E) F**

The cardiac veins run into the coronary sinus, which opens directly into the right atrium. The coronary arteries arise from the ascending aorta at the point where the aorta leaves the left ventricle. The pulmonary artery carries deoxygenated blood to the lungs: after oxygenation the blood returns to the heart via the pulmonary veins.

7.2 **(A) T (B) F (C) T (D) F (E) T**

The circulating blood volume in a 70 kg adult is about 5000 ml (approximately 70 ml/kg body weight). Cardiac output at rest is usually about 5 L/min, rising to 30 L/min with exercise.

7.3 **(A) F (B) F (C) T (D) F (E) F**

AVR is the right arm lead. The standard leads are I, II, III, aVR, aVL and aVF. II, III and aVF are also the 'inferior' leads. The most appropriate lead for pre-hospital monitoring is lead II. The normal paper speed is 25 mm/s.

7.4 **(A) F (B) F (C) F (D) T (E) F**

Pulse oximetry is unreliable in carbon monoxide poisoning as it measures both oxyhaemoglobin and carboxyhaemoglobin, giving a reassuringly false high value. The technique is not affected by skin colour, but may work poorly through metallic nail varnish. Circulation distal to a fracture may be monitored in a finger or toe, but this is not particularly reliable. Cold weather, which reduces distal circulation, will lower the reading on the pulse oximeter.

7.5　(A) T　(B) T　(C) F　(D) T　(E) F

Pulse oximetry measures the saturation of haemoglobin with oxygen, and not levels of carbon dioxide. It cannot, therefore, be used either to monitor alveolar hypoventilation or to assess the progress of respiratory failure. Pulse oximeter readings can be influenced by bright ambient light.

7.6　(A) T　(B) T　(C) F　(D) T　(E) F

Nickel–cadmium batteries require regular conditioning, when the battery is fully discharged before recharging.

7.7　(A) F　(B) F　(C) F　(D) F　(E) T

In adults ventricular fibrillation is the commonest cardiac arrest rhythm, and most cardiac arrests are of primary cardiac origin (usually ischaemic heart disease). The first priority pre-hospital is *safety*. A precordial thump is indicated in witnessed, monitored cardiac arrest when the rhythm is VF, VT or asystole. Opiate overdose results initially in respiratory arrest, but cardiorespiratory arrest invariably follows if there is no appropriate intervention.

7.8　(A) F　(B) F　(C) T　(D) T　(E) T

A precordial thump may deliver up to 20 J of energy. It is delivered over the sternum at the same point as the hand position for external chest compressions. Regular precordial thumps have been used to pace asystolic patients or patients in complete heart block, so called 'fist pacing'. As well as converting VF into sinus rhythm, a precordial thump may convert VF into asystole.

7.9　(A) F　(B) T　(C) F　(D) T　(E) T

The survival rate in asystole is approximately 5%. External pacing is appropriate when the monitor shows P-waves only. Adrenaline 1 mg is given during every cycle of the arrest protocol; 3 mg of atropine is given once only. Very rarely, asystole may revert to sinus rhythm on coughing.

7.10　(A) T　(B) T　(C) T　(D) T　(E) T

All are causes of electromechanical dissociation. Remember: *Think of the causes to begin, and treat them if you want to win.*

7.11   (A) T (B) F (C) T (D) F (E) T

By rendering the blood more alkaline, sodium bicarbonate reduces tissue oxygen dissociation from haemoglobin, and by liberating carbon dioxide it may worsen intracellular acidosis (higher gradient of carbon dioxide across cell membrane, and within the cell CO_2 combines with water to form carbonic acid). The only current indication for sodium bicarbonate is in prolonged arrest when facilities are available for blood gas analysis, and therefore it may be argued that it is not suitable for use outside hospital. Administration of sodium bicarbonate and calcium chloride through the same line will produce calcium carbonate, which is chalk.

7.12   (A) T (B) T (C) T (D) T (E) T

All are risk factors for ischaemic heart disease.

7.13   (A) T (B) T (C) F (D) T (E) F

Immediately following a myocardial infarction (MI), the ECG may be normal in up to 25% of cases. The characteristic ECG marker of an acute myocardial infarction is elevation of the ST segment by more than 2 mm in the corresponding leads. This will not be seen on a rhythm strip pre-hospital unless there is an inferior MI with changes in leads II or III. In general, a 12-lead ECG is needed in the Accident and Emergency Department to make the diagnosis of MI.

Any rhythm is possible immediately following an MI. Bradycardias and heart block are common with inferior infarction (parasympathetic over-activity common), while tachydysrhythmias are common with an anterior infarction (sympathetic overactivity common). Q-waves are a late sign of an infarction, and are often a permanent ECG marker, or 'scar'.

7.14   (A) T (B) F (C) T (D) T (E) T

Headache is a side effect of nitrate-based drugs used in angina, such as GTN.

7.15   (A) T (B) T (C) T (D) F (E) T

Metoclopramide is the antiemetic of choice for the resons given in (C) and (E). The dose of atropine for symptomatic bradycardia (rather than asystole) is 500 µg, repeated as required.

7.16 (A) T (B) T (C) T (D) F (E) T

Pre-hospital thrombolysis should only be given where an agreed protocol has been established. In the UK this is doctor led. Treatment is most effective when given as soon as possible after infarction, and in combination with aspirin (although aspirin administration is *not* time critical, unlike the thrombolysis). Acute peptic ulceration, not a previous history of peptic ulceration, is an absolute contraindication.

7.17 (A) T (B) T (C) T (D) T (E) T

The pain of dissecting aortic aneurysm may be very similar to that of myocardial infarction; the characteristic tearing pain is rare. Furthermore, depending on the location of the dissection, the coronary arteries may be obstructed resulting in true myocardial infarction. Paraplegia may result from obstruction of the spinal arteries. A past history of hypertension is a feature of both myocardial infarction and aortic aneurysm, and cannot be used to discriminate between the two.

7.18 (A) T (B) T (C) T (D) T (E) T

All are causes of cardiac tamponade

7.19 (A) T (B) T (C) F (D) F (E) T

The correct pre-hospital treatment for junctional tachycardia is a vagal manoeuvre followed by rapid transport to hospital where the first line treatment is adenosine. Adenosine is a safe drug in narrow complex tachycardia as it has a very short half-life (less than 10 seconds, rapidly metabolized by red blood cells). Although adenosine is not currently used by ambulance services in the UK, it is a drug that may be considered to add in the future. The treatment for second-degree heart block with cardiovascular compromise is atropine. Synchronous DC shock or lignocaine are appropriate treatments for VT with a pulse, but a conscious patient requires intravenous sedation before a DC shock can be administered. Pulseless VT is treated as VF.

7.20   (A) T (B) T (C) F (D) T (E) T

Eyeball pressure, carotid sinus massage, Valsalva manoeuvre and the diving reflex (ice on the face) all cause slowing of the heart by stimulating the vagus nerve. Eyeball pressure is not recommended, as it may result in a retinal detachment. The diving reflex is virtually vestigial in man, but it may work in infants. Carotid sinus massage should not be performed for more than 5–10 seconds, and only one side at a time, lest the carotid artery is sent into spasm. All of these manoeuvres work best in the young (<40 years), and in the recumbent position.

SHORT ANSWERS

7.21   The figure below shows the cardiac action potential.

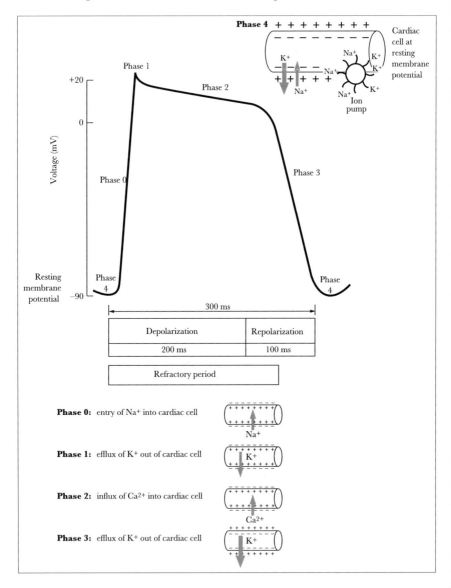

When an electrical depolarization signal reaches the myocardial cell, the following sequence of events occurs:

1. Sodium channels in the membrane open
2. Sodium ions (positively charged) rush into the cell (negatively charged)
3. *This constitutes the QRS complex, and myocardial muscle contraction*
4. Potassium channels open
5. Potassium ions (positively charged) rush out of the cell
6. *This constitutes the T-wave, and myocardial muscle repolarization*
7. The cell is relaxed until the next depolarization signal

7.22 The figure below shows the cardiac conducting system.

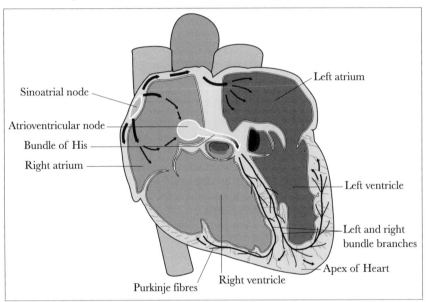

Sinoatrial node

Atrioventricular node

Bundle of His

Right atrium

Left atrium

Left ventricle

Left and right bundle branches

Apex of Heart

Purkinje fibres

Right ventricle

7.23 The diagnosis of pulmonary embolism is made in only 25% of cases before death. This means that it is both difficult to diagnose, and has a very high mortality. Pulmonary embolism (PE) occurs when a thrombus (clot) that has formed in the leg or pelvis becomes dislodged and is conveyed to the lungs. Depending on the size of the thrombus, it may wedge in a main pulmonary artery or in a subsidiary arteriole. The result is a failure to oxygenate blood, increased pressure within the pulmonary artery circuit (pulmonary hypertension), straining of the right ventricle and a failure of the heart to work as an effective pump. The causes of the thrombus are:

1. Abnormalities in the blood vessel (damaged vessel wall)
2. Increased coagulability of blood
3. Obstruction to venous return from the legs or pelvis

Conditions that are associated with venous thrombosis are:

- Pregnancy (pelvic vein obstruction)
- Peri-operative period (venous obstruction during operation; inactivity; increased coagulability of blood)
- Lower limb and pelvic fractures (venous obstruction from secondary oedema; inactivity)
- Carcinoma (pelvic vein compression, e.g. with bowel carcinoma)

Pre-hospital diagnosis is based on recognizing the pattern of clinical features. A mild to moderate PE may produce shortness of breath, chest pain, dizziness and palpitations. A severe PE may cause marked chest pain, hypotension, cough with haemoptysis, marked tachycardia and ultimately cardiac arrest (often in electromechanical dissociation). There may be features of a deep vein thrombosis in the leg (swollen, hot, tender calf muscle), but these are often absent.

The pre-hospital management is:

- Maintain a clear airway
- Give high-flow supplemental oxygen
- Monitor cardiac rhythm, and treat life-threatening dysrhythmias
- Obtain intravenous access
- Give intravenous analgesia where available and required (e.g., nalbuphine)

PICTURE QUIZ

7.24   This figure shows the normal ECG complex. The *P-wave* represents atrial contraction (depolarization). The *PR interval* is the time between atrial and ventricular contraction and is normally less than 0.2 seconds (5 small squares); when prolonged it is called *first-degree heart block*, which is common after myocardial infarction but requires no treatment other than observation. The *QRS complex* (R, first positive deflection after P; Q, a negative deflection between R and P; S, negative deflection after R) represents ventricular contraction and normally lasts less than 0.1 seconds (2.5 small squares); it is prolonged when atrial depolarization is conducted to one of the ventricles with bundle branch block (the second ventricle is then stimulated by wave of depolarization spreading from first ventricle). The *T-wave* represents ventricular repolarization (atrial repolarization is not seen on the ECG). The *ST segment* is usually isoelectric (neither depressed or elevated from the baseline); it is elevated in myocardial infarction and pericarditis, and is depressed in myocardial ischaemia.

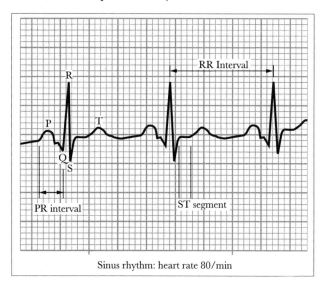

Sinus rhythm: heart rate 80/min

7.25 The rhythms are:

(a) Supraventricular tachycardia

(b) Sinus bradycardia

(c) Second-degree Mobitz type 2 heart block (Wenkebach phenomenon)

(d) Ventricular tachycardia

7.26 The screen is technically showing 'asystole'; however it is also showing that it is reading from the paddles. A defibrillator should be set to default to leads or paddles depending on which method of monitoring will be used first, but if the paddles are not on the chest then paddle mode will display no electrical activity (asystole). A further clue is that 'electrical' asystole (lead fault, or wrong mode selected) will appear as a completely straight line; 'physiological' asystole tends to produce a slowly undulating baseline.

The first actions are:

- Check the patient: establish cardiac arrest
- Check the defibrillator is in the correct mode (leads/paddles) for the monitoring you are performing
- If leads is selected, check all leads are attached
- If there is a gain switch on the monitor, turn it up

All rhythms may appear as 'asystole' if the gain is turned right down.

CASE HISTORY

This patient is hypothermic and in ventricular fibrillation, which is often resistant to treatment until the core temperature is above 30°C. Importantly, VF can be precipitated in the hypothermic patient by careless handling, or rough endotracheal intubation.

The priorities are the same for all patients: *Safety–ABC.* Do not become a casualty yourself. Drowning may have resulted from a fall into the water, or there may have been hyperflexion of the cervical spine on diving: *a cervical spine injury should always be presumed until excluded in hospital.*

The process of hypothermia is arrested and rewarming started by:

- Removal of wet clothing, and drying the body
- Warm blankets
- Infusion of warm intravenous fluid

Intravenous fluid should be given cautiously, unless there is associated hypovolaemia from injury, as fluids are poorly tolerated by the hypothermic patient, with resultant pulmonary oedema.

Although no absolute guidelines exist for the management of ventricular fibrillation in hypothermia, an element of common sense may dictate that where three cycles of the VF protocol have been completed (total of 12 shocks) and the patient is still in VF with a core temperature less than 30°C, then the patient should be rewarmed to >30°C before further shocks are given.

CHEST AND ABDOMINAL TRAUMA

Refer to Chapters 20, 23 and 24 of
Emergency Care: A Textbook for Paramedics.

MULTIPLE CHOICE

8.1 **The immediately life-threatening chest injuries are:**

A. Flail chest

B. Cardiac contusion

C. Tension pneumothorax

D. Cardiac tamponade

E. Pulmonary contusion

8.2 **The following are signs of a tension pneumothorax:**

A. Absent breath sounds on the same side

B. Reduced breath sounds on the opposite side

C. Deviated trachea to the opposite side

D. Tachypnoea

E. Hypotension

8.3 **The following are signs of a massive haemothorax:**

A. Amplified breath sounds on the same side

B. Deviated trachea to the opposite side

C. Distended neck veins

D. Dullness to percussion

E. Reduced chest movement on the same side

8.4 The following are true of chest injuries:

A. Pulmonary contusion is a common fatal chest injury

B. Chest injuries are a more important cause of death than head injuries

C. A tension pneumothorax produces a hyperinflated poorly moving hemithorax

D. A sucking chest injury refers to the noise at the mouth produced by deep, rapid breathing

E. Intrathoracic bowel from a ruptured diaphragm may be clinically mistaken for a pneumothorax

8.5 Concerning an open pneumothorax:

A. The treatment of choice is to cover with a water-tight dressing, sealed on three sides

B. There may be no effective ventilation

C. Air may preferentially move in and out of the chest through the hole in the chest wall

D. Blunt trauma is the characteristic cause

E. The treatment of choice is to seal the wound completely and immediately decompress the chest

8.6 In a patient with suspected cardiac tamponade from a stab wound to the chest, and who is 10 minutes from hospital by road:

A. Rapid intravenous infusion pre-hospital has been shown to save lives

B. Needle pericardiocentesis by an accompanying immediate care doctor may be life-saving if 20 ml of blood are aspirated

C. The knife should be removed if it is still in place

D. The patient should be gently rolled to check for wounds on the back

E. The patient should be frisked for weapons

8.7 These statements about a flail chest are true:

A. It is the abnormal chest movement that causes the greatest respiratory compromise

B. The sternum may be flail

C. Pain relief can be adequately provided with Entonox

D. The flail may not be apparent for some hours

E. A characteristic mechanism is a kick from a horse

8.8   Concerning abdominal trauma:

A.   It is important that the paramedic identifies the organ that may be damaged

B.   Intra-abdominal bleeding may be masked in spinal injury

C.   Abdominal girth is a useful measure to detect intra-abdominal bleeding

D.   The risk of liver injury with fractured lower ribs on the right is 10%

E.   The risk of spleen injury with fractured lower ribs on the left is 20%

8.9   Concerning the MAST suit (Military Anti-shock Trousers; or Pneumatic Anti-shock Garment, PASG):

A.   Any of the segments may be inflated individually

B.   The suit works by increasing peripheral vascular resistance

C.   It is ideal for bilateral fractures of the lower limbs

D.   It must always be deflated slowly

E.   The abdominal segment is contraindicated in advanced pregnancy

8.10   Reliable signs of intra-abdominal injury include:

A.   Reduced bowel sounds

B.   Increasing abdominal girth

C.   Abdominal wall tenderness

D.   Abdominal rigidity

E.   Imprint bruising

8.11   The following may mask the physical signs of abdominal injury:

A.   Alcohol

B.   Multiple injuries

C.   Obesity

D.   Previous abdominal surgery

E.   Diabetes

8.12   Causes of cardiogenic shock include:

A.   Pulmonary embolism

B.   Flail chest

C.   Myocardial infarction

D.   Cardiac contusion

E.   Fluid overload

8.13   The following may produce difficulties in the assessment of a shocked patient:

A.   Beta-blockers

B.   Fitness

C.   Advanced age

D.   Chest injury

E.   Advanced pregnancy

8.14   Features of neurogenic shock include:

A.   Pale, cold peripheries

B.   Hypotension

C.   Bradycardia

D.   Delayed capillary refill

E.   Difficult vascular access

SHORT ANSWERS

8.15   Give an account of the injury mechanisms following blunt trauma to the abdomen.

8.16   List the five life-threatening chest injuries and their pre-hospital treatment.

8.17   List the clinical features of shock and explain why they are unreliable in isolation, and why they may be difficult to elicit.

PICTURE QUIZ

8.18 Discuss the priorities in the management of this patient, and the potential injuries that may be present.

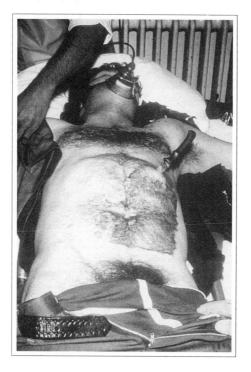

CHEST AND ABDOMINAL TRAUMA

MULTIPLE CHOICE

8.1 (A) T (B) F (C) T (D) T (E) F

Cardiac tamponade, tension pneumothorax and flail chest are three of the five life-threatening chest conditions. The others are an open pneumothorax (sucking chest wound) and massive haemothorax. Outside hospital a flail chest is best managed by appropriate patient positioning (sitting the patient up if possible and applying manual pressure to restrict the paradoxical movement), high-flow oxygen and rapid transport.

Tension pneumothorax is commonly associated with major chest injuries, particularly when positive pressure ventilation is applied, either via a bag-valve-mask or an endotracheal tube. Urgent needle decompression is required, which can be provided at the scene by paramedics of some UK ambulance services, or by an immediate care doctor.

Cardiac contusion usually manifests after a few hours. It is bruising of the heart from direct injury, and may produce dysrhythmias or even cardiogenic shock (pump failure).

Lung contusion is commonly associated with blunt trauma, often with overlying rib fractures in adults. There is haemorrhage into the alveoli and oedema. The affected lung is stiff and does not allow adequate gas exchange. Overtransfusion will worsen a pulmonary contusion.

8.2 (A) T (B) F (C) T (D) T (E) T

The signs of a tension pneumothorax are absent breath sounds on the affected side, plus an increased percussion note (increased resonance). This is because the lung is completely collapsed and the pleural cavity is filled with air. There should be no affect on the breath sounds on the opposite side. As a late feature the trachea deviates to the opposite side. The ensuing hypoxia results in tachypnoea. A reduced venous return and restrictive effect on the heart results in hypotension and tachycardia. Other features are a raised jugular venous pulse (distended neck veins, but not if the patient is hypovolaemic), and a decreasing level of consciousness that reflects the hypoxia.

8.3   (A) F (B) F (C) F (D) T (E) T

A significant amount of blood in one side of the chest is suggested by reduced air entry and dullness to percussion. The trachea is almost always central. Neck veins are usually flat owing to volume loss, and the patient will be in class II or III hypovolaemic shock. In hospital a chest drain is required, and emergency surgical treatment may be needed to stop the bleeding (although it often stops itself if it has arisen from an intercostal vessel). It is essential to have intravenous fluids running before the chest drain is inserted, as bleeding will restart once the haemothorax starts draining.

8.4   (A) T (B) F (C) T (D) F (E) T

Pulmonary contusion is the commonest fatal chest injury following blunt chest trauma, in those who survive the immediate post-injury period (when great vessel disruption is a common cause of death).

Tension pneumothorax produces a hemithorax (one side of the chest) which does not move and may appear overinflated. It is hyper-resonant (sounds like a drum) to percussion and breath sounds cannot normally be heard.

A sucking chest wound describes the movement of air through a chest wall wound during inspiration and expiration. When the wound is more than two-thirds the diameter of the trachea, air will preferentially be drawn through the wound (shorter distance than following the trachea and bronchi), which results in virtually no true ventilation.

Diaphragmatic rupture usually follows blunt trauma where there is herniation of abdominal organs into the chest. This presents as shortness of breath, reduced air entry and a resonant hemithorax (often mistaken for a pneumothorax). The commonest site of rupture is on the left, at the central tendon of the diaphragm.

8.5   (A) T (B) T (C) T (D) F (E) F

An open pneumothorax should be identified in the primary survey. The wound should be sealed on three sides with a square waterproof dressing. This allows air out of the chest on expiration, but prevents air being drawn into the wound on inspiration. It is not the normal remit of a paramedic to seal the wound and decompress the chest completely, although this would be the treatment of choice in the Accident and Emergency Department.

8.6   (A) F (B) T (C) F (D) F (E) F

Rapid intravenous infusion has been shown to be detrimental when given for penetrating cardiac injuries: 'scoop and run' is the only policy for this injury. Intravenous access may be attempted during transit, but fluids should only be given to maintain the systolic blood pressure at 90–100 mmHg.

A small collection of blood within the pericardial sac will constrict the heart, compromising the ventricular filling and the cardiac output. With a patient *in extremis* as little as 20 ml of blood removed by needle pericardiocentesis can be life saving, but in the absence of an experienced doctor the most appropriate action is rapid transport with a request for the trauma team to be on standby.

A penetrating foreign body should not be removed until the patient is in the operating theatre. The patient should essentially be left undisturbed, and the back examined as part of the secondary survey. It is enough pre-hospital to run a gloved hand under the back to check for any gross bleeding.

It is not generally the paramedic's responsibility to check the patient for weapons. However, never assume that a stabbed or shot patient is an innocent victim. There may have been a two-way exchange, and a hypoxic, confused patient who is armed may confuse you for an assailant.

8.7   (A) F (B) T (C) F (D) T (E) T

Flail chest is a life-threatening condition, mainly because of the under-lying lung contusion rather than the paradoxical movement. A flail segment is two or more ribs fractured in two or more places; alternatively, the whole sternum may be flail. Entonox is contraindicated in chest injuries: if there is a small, undetected pneumothorax, nitrous oxide may rapidly diffuse into this causing it to tension.

Initially muscle spasm may mask the paradoxical movement, and it may only be when the intercostal muscles fatigue that it becomes apparent. This may be some hours after the injury.

8.8   (A) F (B) T (C) F (D) T (E) T

The role of the paramedic is to identify an abdominal injury exists, rather than to make a specific diagnosis. The first sign of a problem may be when the patient shows signs of hypovolaemia, but there is no obvious external blood loss. Otherwise, signs of intra-abdominal injury (distension, tenderness, rigidity) may be apparent on a limited secondary survey, where time permits. Spinal injury may mask intra-abdominal signs, if sensation is lost.

Both the liver (10%) and the spleen (20%) may be damaged with lower rib fractures on the corresponding side. On inspiration, these organs rise inside the bony thorax, and a penetrating injury below the level of the nipple should be presumed to involve the intra-abdominal organs.

8.9   (A) F (B) T (C) F (D) T (E) T

The MAST suit (Military Anti-shock Trousers; or Pneumatic Anti-shock Garment, PASG) was originally developed from the pressure suit worn by high-altitude pilots. It consists of three inflatable compartments: two legs, and an abdominal segment. The leg compartments may be inflated on their own, but the abdominal segment can only be used if both legs are inflated first.

A traction splint is the ideal device for bilateral fractured femurs; bilateral fractured tibiae can be managed in box splints. There is the danger with an inflatable splint of further compromising the circulation of a fractured limb.

The MAST suit is thought to work by a combination of increasing the peripheral vascular resistance and shunting blood from the periphery to the central circulation. It is contraindicated to inflate the abdominal segment in advanced pregnancy, or if there is a ruptured diaphragm, pulmonary oedema or significant continuing bleeding above the diaphragm. It must always be deflated slowly, to avoid a precipitous fall in blood pressure.

8.10   (A) F (B) F (C) F (D) T (E) T

Bowel sounds are unreliable as gut motility is reduced in response to any severe trauma. Abdominal girth is unreliable as the stomach is often distended with air from high-flow oxygen or bag-valve-mask ventilation. Muscle tenderness will be common after minor abdominal wall trauma. Abdominal rigidity is an important sign and implies peritoneal irritation and muscle spasm, particularly from free blood. An imprint sign (tyre, seatbelt, steering wheel) is also often a cutaneous marker of significant intra-abdominal injury: it implies compression of the anterior abdominal wall against something firm, such as the vertebral column, the seat or the road.

8.11 (A) T (B) T (C) T (D) F (E) F

Alcohol may modify pain perception and mask the signs of abdominal injury, particularly tenderness and guarding. Obesity can make abdominal examination very difficult. In the presence of painful multiple injuries, such as a dislocation or long bone fracture, the patient may not complain of abdominal pain.

8.12 (A) T (B) F (C) T (D) T (E) F

Cardiogenic shock may follow direct cardiac 'injury' (myocardial infarction; blunt chest trauma causing myocardial contusion), or be an indirect result of impairment of cardiac function, such as a massive pulmonary embolism.

8.13 (A) T (B) T (C) T (D) F (E) T

Beta-blockers will mask the cardiac response to hypovolaemia, which is to increase the heart rate in response to sympathetic stimulation.

A fit young adult may have a resting pulse of 45–50 per minute, and to raise the pulse to 80 per minute is a significant tachycardia. The physiological changes of class I and class II haemorrhagic shock may, therefore, be missed.

The elderly are less able to compensate for volume loss by virtue of a higher incidence of pre-existing disease.

In advanced pregnancy, there is a 50% increase in maternal circulating blood volume. The characteristic physiological signs of hypovolaemia are therefore very late to appear, when deterioration may be precipitous.

8.14 (A) F (B) T (C) T (D) F (E) F

Neurogenic shock is a result of loss of sympathetic control and characteristically produces hypotension, warm peripheries and a bradycardia. Vascular access is often easy because of peripheral venous pooling.

SHORT ANSWERS

8.15   Blunt trauma may produce abdominal injuries secondary to *compression*. A sudden rise in intra-abdominal pressure may rupture a loop of bowel, or cause a diaphragmatic tear. A common cause would be an incorrectly worn seatbelt.

Crush injuries occur when there is direct force applied to the abdominal viscera. The handlebars of a bicycle may crush the duodenum (a fixed structure) against the lumbar spine. Solid fixed viscera such as the liver and spleen are susceptible to crush injury.

Shearing injury occurs when there is a tangential force. Structures at risk are the vascular attachments (pedicles) of solid organs such as the spleen and liver, and the small bowel mesentery. They are commonly seen after rapid deceleration.

Ejection involves a number of forces and mechanisms of injury including compression, crush and shearing. The chance of intra-abdominal injury is high.

8.16   The five life-threatening chest conditions and their pre-hospital treatment are:

1. *Tension pneumothorax:*
   - High-flow oxygen
   - Immediate needle thoracocentesis (if the paramedic does not have this skill, even rapid transport may fail to save the patient)
   - Rapid transport for definitive treatment

2. *Open pneumothorax (sucking chest wound):*
   - High-flow oxygen
   - Square waterproof dressing sealed on three sides
   - Rapid transport
   - Intravenous access during transport

3. *Massive haemothorax:*
   - High-flow oxygen
   - Rapid transport
   - Intravenous access during transport, but fluids should be given only to raise the blood pressure to 90–100 mmHg, otherwise further bleeding will be encouraged

4. *Flail chest:*
   - High-flow oxygen
   - For lateral flail, turn on to the affected side against a pillow
   - Beware of the development of a tension pneumothorax
   - Rapid transport to hospital

5. *Cardiac tamponade:*
   - High-flow oxygen
   - Rapid transport to hospital
   - Leave any penetrating object *in situ*
   - Intravenous access during transport, but intravenous fluids pre-hospital in general have been shown to worsen the prognosis of penetrating cardiac injury
   - A pre-hospital care doctor may attempt needle pericardiocentesis
   - This patient requires a surgeon to be waiting to perform a thoracotomy and oversew the cardiac wound

8.17 The signs of hypovolaemic shock and their reliability are given in the table below.

Clinical sign	Unreliability in assessing shock
Tachycardia	May be caused by anxiety and pain
Pallor	Difficult to see pre-hospital, especially at night
Capillary refill test	Unreliable in cold and dark
Tachypnoea	Unreliable in isolation as may reflect airway obstruction, chest injury, hypovolaemia, anxiety, and pain
Reduced level of response	Also seen in hypoxia from any cause, and in head injury
Blood pressure	Systolic BP alone may not fall until up to 30% of blood volume lost

PICTURE QUIZ

8.18   This patient should be assessed following the ABC guidelines. High-flow
oxygen is given, and a search made for the signs of tension pneumothorax
and cardiac tamponade. In a stab between the nipple and the umbilicus
there may be a thoracic injury, an abdominal injury, or both.

Intravenous access should be established during transport to hospital, but
fluids given only to maintain a blood pressure of 90–100 mmHg.
Aggressive fluid resuscitation promotes further bleeding and worsens the
prognosis.

HEAD AND SPINAL TRAUMA

Refer to Chapters 21, 22 and 26 of *Emergency Care: A Textbook for Paramedics.*

MULTIPLE CHOICE

9.1 **The following are management priorities in isolated head injury:**

A. A primary survey

B. Hyperventilation

C. Immediate CT scan at hospital when the GCS is between 9 and 12

D. Rapid intravenous fluids

E. Steroids

9.2 **Concerning the Glasgow Coma Scale:**

A. Trends are more important than an individual score

B. Eye opening to pain scores 3

C. Incomprehensible sounds scores 2

D. Abnormal flexion scores 2

E. A score <9 requires the airway to be secured by intubation

9.3 **Relating to the anatomy and physiology of the central nervous system:**

A. CSF flows between the arachnoid mater and the dura mater

B. Respiratory and cardiovascular centres are found in the midbrain

C. Pupillary responses are affected by local and central factors

D. An expanding extradural haematoma will often produce ipselateral limb signs

E. The spinal cord ends at the level of the second lumbar vertebra

9.4   Features of an expanding extradural haematoma include:

A.   A high incidence of an associated skull fracture

B.   Hyperthermia

C.   A lucid interval

D.   Priapism

E.   Contralateral pupillary dilatation

9.5   Signs of raised intracranial pressure following head injury are:

A.   Decreasing Glasgow Coma Scale

B.   Hypotension and tachycardia

C.   Tachypnoea

D.   Vomiting

E.   Photophobia

9.6   The following are true in head injury:

A.   Head injuries commonly produce hypotension

B.   All patients require a neurosurgical opinion

C.   Hyperglycaemia is a common sequela

D.   The signs of raised intracranial pressure may be masked by hypovolaemia

E.   It is safe to observe a profoundly drunk patient with a scalp haematoma and a GCS of 7 for 2 hours

9.7   Signs of a spinal cord injury in an unconscious patient are:

A.   Sweating

B.   Warm peripheries

C.   Priapism

D.   Tachycardia

E.   Central cyanosis

9.8   Cerebral oedema:

A.   Is worsened by hypoxia

B.   Is aggravated by injudicious fluid replacement

C.   Is worsened by hypocapnia

D.   Is treated with frusemide pre-hospital

E.   May be exacerbated by prolonged application of a semi-rigid collar

9.9   Risk factors relating to spinal injury include:

A.   Children under 1 year old

B.   Osteoporosis

C.   Rheumatoid arthritis

D.   Muscular dystrophy

E.   Osteoarthritis

9.10   The following are correctly associated:

A.   Pinpoint pupils   Atropine

B.   Dilated pupil   Cataract

C.   Dilated pupil   Eye trauma

D.   Constricted pupils   Adrenaline

E.   Constricted pupils   Tricyclic antidepressant overdose

9.11   Neurogenic shock:

A.   Is due to a loss of parasympathetic function

B.   Normally recovers over 2–3 days

C.   May require atropine for bradycardia

D.   Is more severe the higher the lesion

E.   Is synonymous with spinal shock

9.12   Basal skull fractures:

A.   Are commonly associated with Battle's sign outside hospital

B.   Usually have an associated overlying scalp laceration

C.   May produce a blood and CSF leak from the ear in anterior cranial fossa fractures

D.   Should not be intubated pre-hospital

E.   Have subconjunctival haemorrhage as a consistent feature

9.13   Secondary brain injury can be produced by:

A.   Hypovolaemia

B.   Hypothermia

C.   Overtransfusion

D.   Hypocarbia

E.   Hypoglycaemia

9.14   Concerning facial injuries:

A.   There is an association with cervical spine injury

B.   The incidence of severe injuries has been reduced by wearing seatbelts

C.   Airway obstruction may be relieved by pulling the upper incisors forward

D.   Airway obstruction may be relieved by a tongue suture

E.   Bleeding from the nose means an associated basal skull fracture

SHORT ANSWERS

9.15   List the risk factors that would make you suspect spinal injury.

PICTURE QUIZ

9.16 What is wrong with the way this procedure is being performed?

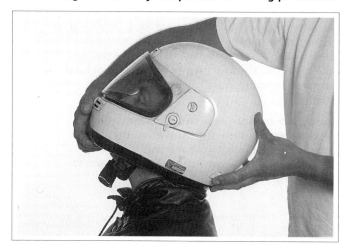

9.17 Explain why the pupil dilates following closed head injury.

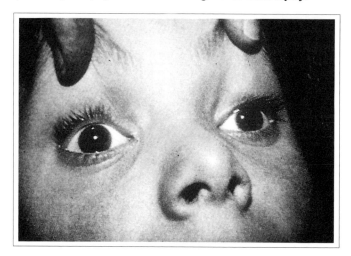

CASE HISTORY

You are called to a street in the town centre at midnight where a scuffle has occurred outside a nightclub. A young couple who are clearly drunk have suffered superficial facial lacerations. They insist on making their own way to the nearby Accident and Emergency department. Lying against a lamp post is a vagrant elderly male well known to the doorman of the nightclub. The vagrant also has superficial facial lacerations and when you attempt to move him he appears unrousable. He smells strongly of alcohol.

- What further information would you require?
- How would you manage the young couple?
- How would you manage the vagrant?
- What is your differential diagnosis for the vagrant?

HEAD AND SPINAL TRAUMA

MULTIPLE CHOICE

9.1   **(A) T (B) F (C) F (D) F (E) F**

As in all trauma victims the priority in management is the primary survey – airway, with control of the cervical spine, breathing with oxygen, circulation with control of external blood loss, disability assessment and limited exposure to identify treatable injuries.

Many head-injured patients are hypoxic owing to airway compromise, and the priority of establishing a clear airway and giving supplemental oxygen cannot be overemphasized.

Hyperventilation may have a role in reducing intracranial pressure by removing excessive carbon dioxide, which is a cerebral vasodilator, but this is generally a hospital intervention after blood gases have been obtained and the head injury assessed by CT scan. The carbon dioxide level in blood must be repeatedly monitored.

CT scanning is not immediately indicated on arrival at hospital until a primary survey has been completed, and hypoxia and hypovolaemia corrected. The main objective is to prevent any secondary brain injury, as the injury sustained at the time of impact is irreversible.

Hypovolaemia is not usually a problem following an isolated head injury, unless there is a severe scalp injury or there is a large intracranial haematoma in a very small infant. An alternative cause should always be sought. Rapid intravenous infusion in an isolated head injury is not indicated and may worsen cerebral oedema.

Steroids have no role in the treatment of cerebral oedema following head injury.

9.2 (A) T (B) F (C) T (D) F (E) T

When using the Glasgow Coma Scale, which is part of the secondary survey, it is important that the patient is regularly reassessed. It is the *trend* that is particularly valuable in guiding emergency management in hospital. An initial GCS of 3 at the scene that improves to 7 in the ambulance and is 10 on arrival at hospital is less worrying than a patient who was fully alert at scene (GCS 15), but who deteriorates to GCS 10 during transport.

Coma is defined as a GCS of 8 or less. Patients in this category require intubation to protect the airway, but this may not be possible pre-hospital unless a doctor is available to administer anaesthetic and muscle relaxant drugs.

9.3 (A) F (B) F (C) T (D) F (E) T

There are three layers of meninges or brain coverings. From the outside inwards, they are the *dura mater*, the *arachnoid mater* and the *pia mater*. Cerebrospinal fluid is found in the subarachnoid space, between the arachnoid and pia mater.

The respiratory and cardiovascular centres are located in the brainstem. With a rise in intracranial pressure and extrusion of the swollen brain there may be direct pressure on these centres.

Pupillary responses can be affected by local and central factors. A direct blow to the eye can cause pupillary dilatation ('traumatic mydriasis'), but in the presence of significant head injury a dilated pupil should always be assumed to reflect an expanding intracranial haematoma on the same side. Limb signs occur on the opposite side of the body to the haematoma.

Anatomically the spinal cord ends and becomes the spinal nerve roots below the first lumbar vertebra.

9.4 (A) T (B) F (C) T (D) F (E) F

An extradural haematoma is commonly associated with a skull fracture. If the patient has a reduced level of response and a skull fracture, the likelihood of a haematoma is 1:4; if the level of response is normal and there is a skull fracture, the likelihood falls to 1:32.

The characteristic history is a transient loss of consciousness, followed by recovery (the 'lucid interval'), then followed by deterioration and death if untreated. Late signs include pupillary dilatation on the same side, together with *bradycardia* and *hypertension* (the *Cushing reflex*). Hyperthermia is seen in brainstem injury and subarachnoid haemorrhage. Priapism (persistent penile erection) is a feature of spinal cord injury.

9.5   (A) T (B) F (C) F (D) F (E) F

A progressive increase in intracranial pressure produces a corresponding fall in the level of response (Glasgow Coma Scale). There is respiratory depression, hypertension and bradycardia. Vomiting is not a specific feature of raised intracranial pressure, and is commonly seen with minor head injury and following a simple skull fracture.

Photophobia is a feature of meningeal irritation. It is not a typical feature of extradural haemorrhage, but is a feature of subarachnoid haemorrhage when there is free blood in the subarachnoid space (also produces neck stiffness).

9.6   (A) F (B) F (C) F (D) F (E) F

Closed head injuries in isolation virtually never produce hypotension from hypovolaemia (unless it is a very large intracranial bleed or a bleed under the scalp, a *cephalhaematoma*, in a very small infant); severe scalp injuries may occasionally cause enough blood loss to cause hypotension. Always look for an alternative cause.

Many thousands of people sustain minor head injuries each year. It is only the moderate and severe head injuries that require a neurosurgical opinion, and clear protocols exist for when a doctor should refer a head-injured patient to a regional neurosurgical unit.

Hypoglycaemia is a common cause of secondary brain injury. The clinical signs of rising intracranial pressure in terms of blood pressure and pulse are opposite to those of hypovolaemia. It is, therefore, possible that hypovolaemia may mask the signs of developing intracranial hypertension.

It is an important maxim never to accept that alcohol is the cause of a reduced level of response when there is an associated head injury. A patient with a GCS of 7 following head injury needs intubating to protect his or her airway, a primary survey to exclude associated injury, a blood glucose check, and a CT scan of the brain.

9.7   (A) F (B) T (C) T (D) F (E) F

Spinal cord injury will abolish the sympathetic nervous system innervation of the heart (causing bradycardia) and the peripheral arterioles (vessels dilate causing peripheral pooling of blood and hypotension). The peripheries are, therefore, warm, unlike in hypovolaemic shock. Sweating is also abolished.

Priapism is due to a loss of parasympathetic control and, following trauma, it is a pathognomonic (absolutely diagnostic) sign of spinal cord injury. Central cyanosis is more likely to be related to an airway or breathing problem.

9.8 (A) T (B) T (C) F (D) F (E) T

Cerebral oedema is worsened by hypoxia, hypovolaemia and hypercarbia (excess carbon dioxide). Treatment in hospital may include hyperventilation to reduce the circulating blood carbon dioxide below normal. Important treatment pre-hospital is to recognize and treat hypoxia and hypovolaemia; there is no role for frusemide here. Diuretics (frusemide and mannitol) are used in the hospital treatment of cerebral oedema, but only after consultation with a neurosurgeon.

A semi-rigid collar will increase intracranial pressure by partially obstructing the venous return from the head. This is not important in those who do not have head injury, but in the presence of head injury it may worsen cerebral oedema. It is important, therefore, to clear the cervical spine of injury early in the hospital management so that the collar can be removed.

9.9 (A) F (B) T (C) T (D) F (E) T

Children are very resistant to spinal injury because of the elastic nature of their skeleton. Spinal wedge fractures are a common feature in osteoporotic bones, particularly in the thoracic and lumbar spine. They are often the result of a compressive force. The commonest area for injury is the junction of the thoraco-lumbar spine, as the thoracic spine is relatively fixed and the lumbar spine relatively mobile.

Patients with rheumatoid arthritis may have involvement of the cervical spine. One characteristic feature is weakening and rupture of the odontoid ligament, which holds the peg of C2 in a stable position within the ring of C1. With rupture of this ligament, the peg may move and impinge on the spinal cord. There may additionally be erosive changes in the cervical spine predisposing to subluxation of one vertebra on another.

Muscular dystrophy may predispose to falls, but is not associated with an increased incidence of spinal injury *per se*.

Osteoarthritis in the cervical spine is called *cervical spondylosis*. Part of the problem is a narrowing of the spinal canal with bony ridges; outgrowths of bone (osteophytes) may also impinge on nerve roots. In the elderly it is not uncommon for there to be neurological changes following a fall, although there are no new changes seen on an X-ray.

9.10   (A) F (B) F (C) T (D) T (E) F

Atropine produces pupil dilatation. As *bella donna* it was used by women to make their appearance more seductive. When given in cardiac arrest, it prevents the interpretation of pupillary dilatation as an indication of brain death. Pupil dilatation is also a feature of tricyclic antidepressant overdose, together with tachycardia, and reduced level of response. Malignant tachydysrhythmias may occur including VT.

9.11   (A) F (B) F (C) T (D) T (E) F

Neurogenic shock follows the loss of sympathetic nervous system function (see question 9.7). The higher the spinal cord injury, the greater the chance and severity of neurogenic shock (the sympathetic outflow is between T1 and T12). The characteristic features are bradycardia and hypotension. Following injury hypotension should not be assumed to be a result of spinal shock, and should always initially be treated as hypovol-aemia. The specific treatment of spinal shock will include atropine and other vasopressor drugs (drugs which cause constriction of peripheral arterioles).

Neurogenic shock is not synonymous with spinal shock. Spinal shock refers to when the reflexes are lost below the level of a cord transection. They often return in 2–3 days.

9.12   (A) F (B) F (C) F (D) F (E) F

There are a number of characteristic signs of a basal skull fracture, including:

- Subconjunctival haemorrhage without a visible posterior limit
- Bruising over the mastoid (behind the ear) or *Battle's sign*
- Bleeding or CSF from the ear
- CSF from the nose

Battle's sign will develop after a few hours, and will not be a useful sign in the pre-hospital phase. CSF leak (and blood) from the nose occurs with an anterior cranial fossa fracture; bleeding and CSF leak from the ear occurs with a middle cranial fossa fracture.

There is no contraindication to intubation pre-hospital, if clinically indicated. Nasal airways are not generally recommended because of the risk of introducing the airway into the brain through an anterior cranial fossa fracture.

9.13   (A) T (B) F (C) T (D) F (E) T

Secondary brain injury can be reduced or prevented by adequate maintenance of blood volume and prevention of hypoxia. Overtransfusion will worsen oedema, as will both hypoglycaemia and hyperglycaemia. One treatment of cerebral oedema is to hyperventilate the patient to reduce the circulating carbon dioxide, which is a cerebral vasodilator.

9.14   (A) T (B) T (C) T (D) T (E) F

There is an increased likelihood of a cervical spine injury with severe facial or head injuries. The incidence of severe facial injuries has, however, been significantly reduced by the wearing of seatbelts by the driver and front seat passenger.

Airway obstruction in a *Le Fort* fracture (after René Le Fort, a Parisien anatomist who studied the pattern of facial fractures in cadavers he had mutilated) may occur when the shattered facial skeleton slides posteriorly along the base of the skull. Life-saving treatment would include lifting the face forward by traction on the upper incisors.

With severe disruption to the jaw, airway obstruction may be relieved by a suture placed transversely across the tongue and applying traction to the tongue.

Bleeding from the nose may occur with a fractured base of the skull (anterior cranial fossa), but it is much more common after direct nose injury. Other evidence of a basal skull fracture should be sought (CSF from the nose; blood or CSF from the ear; Battle's sign; racoon eyes).

SHORT ANSWER

9.15   The risk factors that would increase the likelihood of a spinal injury include:

- Pre-existing spinal disease, including osteoarthritis, rheumatoid arthritis, and ankylosing spondylitis.
- History of the incident, particularly road traffic accident, falls > 5 metres, gymnastics, collapsed rugby scrum, horse riding, hang gliding, board diving, weight falling onto the back.

PICTURE QUIZ

9.16 A crash helmet should be removed by two persons, at least one of whom should be trained. It is a skilled technique which risks injury to the cervical cord. The only immediate indication for removal is airway obstruction, when it would be acceptable for a single operator to perform.

9.17 Pupillary dilatation is a reflection of a rise in intracranial pressure. An expanding intracranial mass causes extrusion of the temporal lobe of the brain on the same side, through the narrow gap between the tentorium cerebelli (a fibrous sheet separating the brain from the cerebellum) and the brainstem which pierces a hole through the tentorium. The extruded brain, therefore, presses on the brainstem, squashing the third cranial nerve nucleus. It is this nerve that controls pupil constriction on the same side.

CASE HISTORY

The further information you require includes: is the scene safe for yourself, for bystanders, and for the casualties? A police presence would usually be required. You would also need to know if there were any other casualties, as further ambulances would be needed.

You cannot force a patient into an ambulance, and this young couple should be advised of the importance of seeking medical attention. If there is a friend or relative who is sober, and who can escort them to accident and emergency this would be ideal.

A patient who has been involved in a fight and who is unrousable must be assumed to have a head injury, even though he smells strongly of alcohol. The chance of a head injury is increased in this case as there is evidence of craniofacial trauma (facial lacerations). The airway should be cleared and secured, and supplemental oxygen given. Intubation may be required. Life-threatening breathing injuries should be excluded, as should haemorrhage from any other major laceration (it is possible this man has been stabbed). He is at risk from a spinal injury and should be transferred on to the ambulance cot using a spinal board; a hard collar and head box would be appropriate precautions. Intravenous access may be obtained depending on the proximity to hospital, but for an isolated head injury intravenous fluids would not be required. A blood sugar estimation should be made, and some ambulance services have this facility. Intravenous dextrose would be a more appropriate method of treating hypoglycaemia than intramuscular glucagon, as glucagon may not be effective in a chronic alcoholic who has low liver glycogen stores.

MUSCULO-SKELETAL TRAUMA

Refer to Chapter 25 of
Emergency Care: A Textbook for Paramedics.

MULTIPLE CHOICE

10.1 **The following can directly or indirectly produce airway compromise:**

A. Sterno-clavicular dislocation

B. Rib fractures

C. Hyoid bone fracture

D. Facial fractures

E. Skull fracture

10.2 **The following can be regarded as life-threatening injuries:**

A. Femoral shaft fracture

B. Tibial shaft fracture

C. Pelvic fracture

D. Posterior hip dislocation

E. Cervical spine injury

10.3 **Early complications of long bone fractures that may be detected pre-hospital are:**

A. Fat embolism

B. Acute compartment syndrome

C. Volkman's ischaemic contracture

D. Acute vascular insufficiency

E. Mal union

10.4   Concerning fractures of the shaft of the femur:

A.   They are commonly associated with major blood vessel injury or nerve damage

B.   Blood loss is 1–1.5 litres in closed fractures

C.   They should always be formally immobilized prior to transfer

D.   They are commonly associated with injuries to the ipselateral (same side) knee

E.   In isolation they should be regarded as a major injury

10.5   Concerning shoulder dislocations:

A.   They commonly result from a fall on to an outstretched hand

B.   Posterior dislocation is more common than anterior dislocation

C.   They may be recurrent

D.   They may be associated with nerve damage

E.   They should be reduced at the scene

10.6   The following are true of a fractured neck of femur:

A.   Occurs exclusively in elderly patients

B.   The affected leg often appears short and externally rotated

C.   The fracture can occur prior to falling over

D.   An intravenous infusion should be established

E.   Immobilization may be achieved using a traction splint

10.7   In children who sustain fractures:

A.   Cervical spine fractures are less common than adults

B.   Rib fractures are associated with a greater incidence of significant underlying chest injury

C.   Entonox is contraindicated

D.   Growth plate injuries are common

E.   A fractured femur is a common injury in a road traffic accident

10.8   Pelvic fractures:

A.   Are common in the elderly

B.   May account for unexplained hypovolaemia in the unconscious patient

C.   Are reliably detected by springing the pelvis

D.   May require urgent surgical stabilization

E.   Can be associated with urethral damage

10.9   The following are common fractures in the elderly:

A.   Colles' fracture ('dinner fork' fracture) of the wrist

B.   Humeral shaft

C.   Thoracic vertebra

D.   Calcaneum (heel)

E.   Neck of femur

10.10   Supracondylar fractures of the humerus:

A.   Are most common in adults

B.   Usually occur due to a direct blow

C.   Have a high incidence of nerve and artery associated injury

D.   Are associated with a fracture of the clavicle on the same side

E.   Should be immobilized with the elbow at 90 degrees

10.11   Orthopaedic injuries commonly associated with neurovascular damage are:

A.   Knee dislocation

B.   Rib fracture

C.   Ankle dislocation

D.   Supracondylar fracture of the humerus

E.   Hip prosthesis dislocation

SHORT ANSWERS

10.12   Why is it important to immobilize a long bone fracture?

10.13   Discuss the uses and contraindications of a traction splint.

PICTURE QUIZ

10.14 You arrive at the home of this lady who has slipped on the stairs. Describe your overall management of this patient.

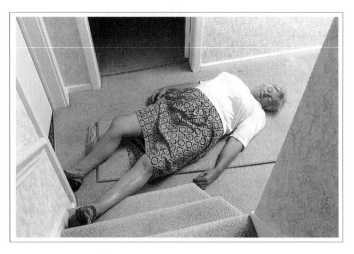

10.15 This boy has fallen off a swing. He has a displaced supracondylar fracture of the humerus. Discuss the management at the scene, and the complications that may develop.

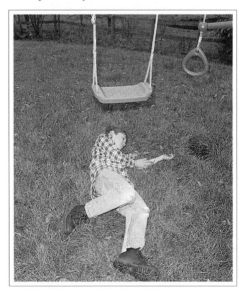

MUSCULO-SKELETAL TRAUMA

MULTIPLE CHOICE

10.1 (A) T (B) F (C) T (D) T (E) T

Fractures of the skull may produce airway compromise both directly owing to bleeding from the base of the skull, and indirectly as a result of an altered level of consciousness. The latter is particularly a problem in those patients with an AVPU scale of P or U, or a Glasgow Coma Scale of 8 or less (the true definition of 'coma').

Facial fractures with posterior displacement of the maxilla (Le Fort fracture) may compromise the airway, but can be treated simply by pulling the face forward with traction on the patient's upper front teeth. Fractures of the mandible may allow the tongue to fall backwards, which may be overcome by sitting the patient forward or rolling him on to his or her side, depending on his or her level of consciousness. The hyoid bone supports the airway above the larynx. It may be injured by a direct blow, after which haemorrhage and oedema can partially obstruct the airway.

Posterior sternoclavicular dislocation can produce airway obstruction which is relieved simply by pulling the clavicle forwards

10.2 (A) T (B) F (C) T (D) F (E) T

Femoral shaft fractures, particularly open (compound) fractures, are associated with severe blood loss. Tibial shaft fractures, even if compound, will rarely be associated with life-threatening blood loss. Fractures of the pelvis can be associated with catastrophic blood loss. High-impact injury causing posterior pelvic ring disruption is particularly dangerous, as the web of vessels that lies in front of the sacrum is often damaged. In some cases in excess of 20 units of blood will be required in the resuscitation. Posterior hip dislocation in isolation is not life-threatening, but it is often caused by impact with the dashboard and this is also a mechanism for femoral shaft fracture – so look for both injuries.

If there is a fracture or dislocation of the cervical spine above C3, this is often incompatible with life. An injury at C3–C5 can cause significant respiratory compromise: remember that the nerve roots *C3,4,5 keep the diaphragm alive*. With an injury immediately below C5, the diaphragm function is intact, but there will be intercostal muscle paralysis. Spinal shock can also coexist, when the muscle tone of large blood vessels is lost resulting in hypotension.

10.3   (A) F (B) T (C) F (D) T (E) F

Following a fracture, fat may escape into the circulation. This may lodge in the lungs, brain and skin, and in combination with the release of biochemical mediators it produces the syndrome of *fat embolism*. In the conscious patient it commonly manifests after a few hours as confusion, shortness of breath, and a petechial (pinpoint bleeding under the skin) rash. It can be prevented in part by adequate resuscitation with the correction of hypoxia and hypovolaemia.

Acute compartment syndrome occurs when a muscle swells within its rigid fibrous compartment sufficiently to obstruct the circulation. Distal pulses are initially present and cannot be used as a reliable sign; pre-hospital, a reduction in the capillary return to the toe, compared to the other side, may be detected. Pain in excess of that associated with the injury (often a fracture) is important. As this syndrome often takes time to develop, it may not be apparent in the pre-hospital phase following injury.

Volkman's ischaemic contracture occurs because of failure to recognize an acute compartment syndrome (or vessel injury) of the forearm, often following a supracondylar fracture of the humerus or dislocated elbow. The result is contraction of the flexor muscles and a 'claw hand'.

Acute vascular insufficiency produces a pale, cold, numb and pulseless distal limb, with severe pain. Again this would occur in the arm following supracondylar fracture or elbow dislocation. With a displaced or angulated fracture, manipulation of the fracture to restore alignment will often restore the distal circulation. This is appropriate pre-hospital, but if dislocation is present, this will be reduced in hospital and the patient should be transported as a priority.

Mal union refers to when the fracture has healed, but in a non-anatomical position.

10.4   (A) F (B) T (C) F (D) T (E) T

The blood loss is often 1–1.5 litres in closed injury, but may be double this if the fracture is compound. The blood loss is a result of damage to the medullary cavity and soft tissues, rather than major blood vessel transection. Damage of the femoral or sciatic nerve is rare. If a patient has continuing airway and breathing problems it would be appropriate to ignore any skeletal injury while rapidly transporting the patient to hospital. Ideally, however, the fracture should be immobilized as this will reduce blood loss and the chance of fat embolism.

Approximately 50% of patients with femoral shaft fractures have associated knee injuries, usually ligamentous affecting the cruciates (inside the knee, stabilizing the knee from moving forwards and backwards) or the collaterals (to each side of the knee, stabilizing the knee from moving side to side).

10.5   (A) T (B) F (C) T (D) T (E) F

Shoulder dislocations can be anterior or posterior, but the vast majority are anterior. Both can occur by falling on to an outstretched hand, but when there is an external rotating force the dislocation is anterior, and when there is an internal rotating force the dislocation is posterior. A direct blow can also cause dislocation.

Extensive damage to the soft tissues around the joint is common, and this predisposes to a recurrent problem. As the brachial plexus, and axillary nerve in particular, are closely associated with the shoulder either may be damaged. Axillary nerve damage is suspected if there is numbness on the outer aspect of the arm.

If a doctor is present at the scene who is expert, for example, a football or rugby team doctor, then reduction is occasionally approriate pre-hospital. Otherwise, the patient should be transported in the most comfortable position for reduction in hospital following X-ray.

10.6   (A) F (B) T (C) T (D) F (E) T

A fractured neck of femur is a common injury in the elderly, more often in women, and is associated with osteoporosis. A small number will give a history of feeling the fracture occur before falling. The characteristic appearance is of a shortened externally rotated leg, but this is not always seen. Blood loss from this injury would very rarely be life-threatening and an intravenous infusion pre-hospital is not routinely indicated. It would be important, of course, to rule out associated injuries sustained in the fall that do require fluid resuscitation pre-hospital.

10.7 (A) T (B) T (C) F (D) T (E) T

The child has a much more elastic skeleton than an adult. With chest injuries the chest wall will deform to a greater extent and intrathoracic organs are more likely to be damaged. Worryingly, there is often not the marker of rib fractures to direct the paramedic or doctor to this underlying injury.

Entonox can be given to children, but compliance is required. A mouthpiece is often more acceptable than a face mask.

The distal end of long bones contain a growth plate (epiphysis) and this is often the point of fracture. With good reduction of any displaced epiphysis it is usual for the bone to grow normally.

Because of the relative height of a child, a femoral fracture is a common injury when hit by the bumper of a car.

Cervical spine injuries are less common than in adults, and when they do occur they are more often the upper cervical spine, rather than the mid-cervical fractures seen in adults.

10.8 (A) T (B) T (C) F (D) T (E) T

Fractures of the pelvis can occur at any age. They are associated with high-impact injuries, such as a road traffic accident, but in the elderly a lesser degree of force such as a simple fall may be enough to fracture a pubic ramus (one of the four struts of the pelvis at the front). Severe pelvic fractures are often associated with genitourinary injury. Urethral injury should be suspected if there is blood at the urethral opening, or a scrotal haematoma. Diagnosis is difficult at the scene. Pelvic spring will detect gross instability, but it is painful, and may precipitate further bleeding.

Prompt transfer to hospital with severe pelvic injury is life-saving. Catastrophic blood loss is only controlled by surgical stabilization of the pelvis.

Unexplained hypovolaemia may be a result of blood loss into the pelvis, abdomen, chest, around a missed long bone fracture or the retro-peritoneum (around the kidneys).

10.9 (A) T (B) F (C) T (D) F (E) T

Colles' fractures, thoracic vertebral fractures, femoral neck fractures and humeral *neck* fractures occur commonly in the elderly as a result of osteoporosis. They are often the result of trivial trauma. Humeral shaft fractures in the elderly occur following direct injuries. Fractures of the calcaneum (heel) are uncommon, and are usually seen in people who fall from a height on to their heels.

10.10 (A) F (B) F (C) T (D) F (E) F

The majority of supracondylar fractures occur in children, and follow a fall on to the outstretched hand. As major nerves and blood vessels are closely associated, there is a high incidence of nerve and vessel injury. The brachial artery may be caught between the bone ends, or stretched over the displaced fracture segment. The limb should be splinted in the position found. In children, 2–3% have an associated wrist fracture. There is no correlation with fractures of the clavicle.

10.11 (A) T (B) F (C) T (D) T (E) T

Knee dislocation may be associated with popliteal vessel injury. Ankle dislocation can impair skin perfusion on the dorsum of the foot. A supracondylar fracture of the humerus may impinge on the brachial artery and, if uncorrected, may lead to flexor muscle necrosis in the forearm. A dislocated hip (posterior) may damage the sciatic nerve.

SHORT ANSWERS

10.12 Long bone fractures should be immobilized, unless continued management of a difficult airway and ventilation prevents further progression along the primary survey. Splintage is part of resuscitation because it reduces blood loss.

Immobilization of a fracture achieves:

- Reduction of pain
- Reduction of blood loss (by 20–30% with femoral shaft fractures)
- Reduction of tension on soft tissues, including nerves, vessels, the skin and muscle
- Reduction of the risk of fat embolism
- Reduction of the risk of secondary injury, such as vessels and nerves, during handling and transportation
- Aids the handling of the patient during transport

10.13 Traction splints reduce pain by immobilization, and reduce blood loss by the mechanical effect of changing the swollen, spherical thigh into an ovoid, which holds less fluid. Secondary damage is prevented and patient handling is improved. A Sager splint can immobilize both fractured femurs in the same splint, while still fitting on the ambulance cot.

Contraindications include a major pelvic fracture, as the pelvis provides the countertraction for all of these splints. Fractures around the knee, in particular the supracondylar fracture, should not be placed in traction as the distal fragment tends to tip backwards and may then impinge on the vessels behind the knee (popliteal vessels). Similarly, a knee dislocation should not be placed in traction, as vascular injury may be exacerbated, apart from it being excruciatingly painful.

10.14 After establishing that the area is safe, assess the patient's ABC and level of response. Treat life-threatening problems as you find them. You observe that the right leg appears shortened and externally rotated, consistent with a fractured neck of femur. This should be immobilized for transport, which is often neglected. A brief history will exclude any obvious precipitating cause for the fall. Your observation of a 'loose carpet' recorded in the medical notes may prompt a visit from social services before discharge, preventing a recurrence of a fall.

10.15 Safety is always the first priority. A primary survey will then exclude other more important life-threatening injuries. Circulation should be assessed in the injured limb (is there a radial pulse?) as should nerve function (can the child gently move his or her fingers, and can he or she feel light touch on the fingers?). If a pulse cannot be felt, the child must be transported as a priority. Immobilization is in the position you find the limb.

Complications of severely displaced supracondylar fractures include damage to the brachial artery and associated nerves, with subsequent development of a compartment syndrome in the forearm. If this goes unrecognized, the muscles of the forearm will die, fibrose and contract, resulting in a *Volkman's ischaemic contracture.*

SPECIAL INCIDENTS I

Refer to Chapters 28, 29, 30 and 41 of
Emergency Care: A Textbook for Paramedics.

MULTIPLE CHOICE

11.1   At the scene of a bomb:

A.   Secondary devices are common

B.   The first priority is your own safety

C.   A dead body at risk of further damage from fire should be moved

D.   Radios should not be used until authority is given from the police

E.   The army bomb disposal unit are in overall control

11.2   The following are true of injuries from a bomb:

A.   Blast lung is common in survivors

B.   Fragments are the commonest cause of injury

C.   Acute deafness may occur

D.   Avulsed limbs must accompany the patient to hospital and are often amenable to reimplantation

E.   The blast wind may be responsible for deceleration injuries

11.3   In gunshot injury:

A.   The degree of injury is more dependent on the mass of the bullet than the speed at which it is travelling

B.   Bullets from a handgun only produce low-energy transfer wounds

C.   A shotgun fired at 3 metres is generally less lethal than a handgun

D.   The size and position of external wounds correlates well with internal injury

E.   Bone may form secondary fragments

11.4   The following suggest an upper airway burn:

A.   Hoarse voice

B.   Singed hair

C.   Oedema of the tongue

D.   Coughing up soot

E.   Blistering on the lips

11.5   Concerning carbon monoxide poisoning:

A.   This may occur insidiously

B.   It usually produces a 'cherry red' discoloration of the skin

C.   Pulse oximetry is unreliable

D.   The specific treatment is oxygen

E.   A patient who recovers from unconsciousness at the scene should receive hyperbaric oxygen

11.6   Functions of the skin include:

A.   A barrier to infection

B.   Control of temperature

C.   Detection of the nature of the environment

D.   Prevention of water loss

E.   Maintenance of body shape

11.7   Following a 30% partial thickness burn:

A.   A child will require relatively more fluid replacement than in an adult

B.   Fluid loss is maximal in the first 24 hours

C.   In an adult the patient will require transfer to a Burns Unit

D.   Silver sulphadiazine cream should not be applied to soothe the burn before transfer

E.   'Cling film' can be used as a dressing

11.8   Concerning chemical burns:

A.   The burn should be liberally irrigated

B.   'Cling film' makes the best dressing

C.   Hydrochloric acid burns are treated with calcium gluconate

D.   Bitumen burns are treated with butter

E.   Acids produce relatively more damage than alkalis

11.9   The following definitions are correct:

A.   A *laceration* is a breach in the skin from a sharp object

B.   A *cut* is a breach in the skin from a blunt object

C.   A *contusion* is a collection of subcutaneous blood

D.   An *abrasion* is a loss of the outer layers of the skin

E.   A *closed wound* produces internal injury without breach of the skin

11.10   Factors affecting wound healing include:

A.   Age of the patient

B.   Age of the wound

C.   Wound infection

D.   Presence of a foreign body

E.   Exposure to ionizing radiation

11.11   Concerning electrocution:

A.   The greatest damage occurs to tissues with a low resistance

B.   DC current is more dangerous than AC current

C.   The size of the skin burn correlates well with the degree of tissue injury

D.   With lightning the majority of the current will pass over the outside of the body

E.   Respiratory arrest is the commonest cause of death

SHORT NOTES

11.12   List the criteria for transfer to a Burns Unit.

11.13   Discuss the estimation of burn area in an adult and child.

11.14 How does a high-energy transfer missile wound differ from a low-energy transfer missile wound?

PICTURE QUIZ

11.15 What are the priorities on arrival at the scene of this bombing?

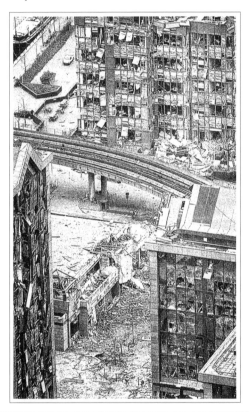

CASE HISTORY

You attend the scene of a reported shooting outside a public house on Saturday night. As you approach you see that everyone is running away from the scene and there is a man on the pavement with a bloodstained shirt. What are your actions?

SPECIAL
INCIDENTS I

MULTIPLE CHOICE

11.1 (A) T (B) T (C) T (D) T (E) F

Secondary terrorist devices are common, and radios should not be used at the scene until a sweep has been made for such devices – in case one is radio-controlled. The civilian police will be in control of a bomb scene, not the army bomb disposal unit.

11.2 (A) F (B) T (C) T (D) F (E) T

Blast lung (widespread haemorrhage into the alveoli) is seen in only 0.6% of survivors of bomb injury. The commonest cause of injury following a bomb is fragmentation, but other mechanisms are the blast wave, the blast wind, burns, crush and psychological injury. The blast wind carries fragments (secondary fragments, e.g. wood, glass, stone); it may also carry the body and produce deceleration injury on impact with a solid object. In addition, the blast wind is responsible for avulsive amputations. These avulsed limbs are rarely amenable for reimplantation surgery, as opposed to limbs amputated by a 'guillotine' mechanism.

11.3 (A) F (B) F (C) F (D) F (E) T

The velocity of a missile is a greater determinant of its potential energy than its mass. Doubling the mass doubles the energy available, but doubling the velocity increases the available energy by four times. However, it is no longer appropriate to consider gunshot wounds simply in terms of 'high velocity' or 'low velocity', but rather in terms of the degree of energy transfer. The amount of energy transferred depends on the retardation of the missile, which in turn is dependent upon the density and elasticity of the tissues, and on missile factors such as deformability. Pieces of shattered bone can act as secondary fragments.

11.4   (A) T (B) F (C) T (D) T (E) T

A hoarse voice is a late sign, and implies laryngeal oedema and impending airway obstruction. Singed *nasal* hair may suggest an upper airway burn, as may carbonaceous sputum (coughing up soot), or a history of fire in an enclosed space.

11.5   (A) T (B) F (C) T (D) T (E) T

Carbon monoxide poisoning may be insidious, such as that which arises from a faulty gas appliance. The textbook cherry-red appearance of the skin is very rare: pallor is more commonly seen. Pulse oximetry is unreliable as it cannot differentiate between normal oxygenated haemoglobin and haemoglobin bound to carbon monoxide. A falsely high oximetry reading may fool the paramedic into thinking that supplemental oxygen is not required, which is the specific antidote for this poison.

Hyperbaric oxygen should be considered for all patients who have been unconscious following carbon monoxide poisoning. This part of the history is, therefore, very relevant at the hospital. It is also considered if the patient is pregnant, has any abnormal neurological signs or has a carboxyhaemoglobin level exceeding 20% in Accident and Emergency. Hyperbaric chamber facilities are very limited, and there will invariably need to be a secondary transfer to an appropriate facility.

11.6   (A) T (B) T (C) T (D) T (E) F

The skeleton is responsible for the body shape, not the skin.

11.7   (A) T (B) T (C) T (D) T (E) T

Children have a larger surface area to volume ratio and have relatively greater fluid requirements following a burn. Creams of any description are not recommended if there is to be a secondary transfer, as these will have to be removed to reassess the burn. 'Cling film' makes a good first-aid and transfer dressing as it allows continued inspection of the wound, it is non-adhesive, it provides an antibacterial screen and it is cheap. The indications for transfer to a Burns Unit are listed in question 11.12.

11.8 **(A) T (B) F (C) F (D) T (E) F**

The immediate treatment of a chemical burn is to remove contaminated clothing and to use copious irrigation. An occlusive dressing, such as 'Cling film', should only be applied to such a burn if it is certain that all the chemical has been removed, otherwise any residual may be trapped. Hydro*fluoric* acid burns are treated with calcium gluconate gel. Hot bitumen (tar) is emulsified by butter. Although such treatment may appear somewhat medieval, butter on a gauze dressing can have a remarkable effect in removing tar after a few minutes. The alternatives are all painful, largely ineffective and rarely indicated.

11.9 **(A) F (B) F (C) T (D) T (E) T**

A *laceration* is a breach in the skin from a blunt object. A *cut* is a breach in the skin from a sharp object. This simple differentiation is all important when the paramedic is asked to provide a police statement for the Coroner's court. Was it actually a cut sustained by the defendant's knife, or was it a laceration from some other blunt trauma?

11.10 **(A) T (B) T (C) T (D) T (E) T**

Other factors affecting wound healing are pre-existing disease (such as diabetes, or AIDS) and drugs (such as steroids or immunosuppressants).

11.11 **(A) F (B) F (C) F (D) T (E) T**

The size of an electrical burn can be very deceptive. Small cutaneous full-thickness burns may mask significant underlying tissue necrosis.

SHORT NOTES

11.12 The criteria for transport to a burns unit are:

- Partial-thickness burn >10% in children or the elderly, or >20% in adults (15–65 years)
- Full-thickness burn >5%
- Chemical burn
- Electrical burn
- Burns of special areas (eyelids; genitalia)

In general, patients will not be transferred directly from the scene to a Burns Unit, but will be a secondary transfer from the first receiving hospital.

11.13 There are a number of ways to estimate the burn surface area:

- The palm of the patient represents 1% of the body surface area, in adults or children
- The *Rule of nines* applies to adults (9% each upper limb; 18% each lower limb; 18% front of torso; 18% back of torso; 9% head; 1% genitalia), but *not* to infants (head 19%; proportionately smaller limbs) or children (head and each lower limb 14%)
- The Lund and Browder chart is a body surface area map corrected for age

11.14 A low-energy transfer wound produces injury by crushing and laceration. The degree of injury will depend on the size and shape of the missile and through which organs it passes. The wound track produced by the missile is known as the *permanent cavity*.

A high-energy transfer wound produces a permanent cavity, but also produces a *temporary cavity*. Here the tissues continue to move away from the wound track for several milliseconds after the missile has passed through. The cavity then collapses and sucks in debris from the wound surface. Structures remote from the wound track can be severely damaged, and this is more common when the missile passes through high-density tissue which increases the retardation of the missile and the energy transfer.

PICTURE QUIZ

11.15 The priorities at the scene of a bomb are:

- *Command*: take charge of the situation, and any bystanders
- *Safety*: yourself (do not approach an incident unless you are sure it is safe to do so), the scene (park to protect the scene and prevent others from entering the scene; evacuate the area), the casualties
- *Communication*: inform control of the situation, but avoid the radio until the scene is cleared of secondary devices
- *Assessment*: of the number and severity of casualties
- *Triage*: sort the casualties into priorities for treatment
- *Treatment*: provide 'ABC' support
- *Transport*: move patients to hospital

CASE HISTORY

This is your judgement call. You must decide whether it is safe to
approach the casualty with caution, or whether you must wait for the
police to secure the scene.

In either case *never* assume the casualty is an innocent party. He or she
may also be armed. A casualty who has lost blood will be hypoxic, and a
hypoxic casualty is often confused and aggressive. Do not allow the
situation that an armed casualty mistakes you for an assailant, so *frisk all
casualties who have been shot or stabbed.*

Once the scene is safe, the casualty will be stabilized along ABC lines.
Rapid transport is absolutely essential in penetrating chest trauma. Recent
studies have suggested that the mortality in these cases is *increased* by
aggressive fluid resuscitation pre-hospital or in the Accident and Emergency Department. The only treatment that will save life with massive
blood loss or cardiac injury is surgery, and patients must get to the operating theatre as quickly as possible.

SPECIAL INCIDENTS II

Refer to Chapters 38, 39, 40, 42 and 43 of
Emergency Care: A Textbook for Paramedics.

MULTIPLE CHOICE

12.1 The following are true:

A. Hypothermia is a core temperature of $<35°C$

B. Severe hypothermia is a core temperature below $32°C$

C. Natural wool is a poor protector against heat loss

D. The normal body temperature is $36–38°C$

E. Careless handling of hypothermia victims may precipitate VF

12.2 Factors increasing heat loss include:

A. Contact with dense materials

B. Wind chill

C. Large surface area:volume ratio

D. Wet clothing

E. Fatigue

12.3 Space blankets:

A. Must be placed outside a normal blanket

B. Protect mainly against conductive heat loss

C. May prevent absorption of heat from the sun

D. Are ineffective against convective loss

E. Are an effective method of active rewarming

12.4   The following are generally accepted with regard to hypothermia:

A.   Loss of coordination begins at 32°C

B.   The risk of spontaneous VF begins at 30°C

C.   Shivering is lost at 30°C

D.   Defibrillation may be ineffective

E.   Atrial fibrillation may occur below 34°C

12.5   The effects of hypothermia include:

1.   Hypotension

2.   Mild confusion

3.   Slurred speech

4.   Unconsciousness

5.   Asystole

As the temperature falls, in which order do these generally occur?

A.   1–3–2–5–4

B.   2–1–3–5–4

C.   1–2–5–3–4

D.   3–2–1–5–4

E.   2–3–4–1–5

12.6   The following are true:

A.   20% of deaths due to drowning occur in children <5 years

B.   10 ml of water per kg body weight if inhaled may be fatal

C.   The mechanism of death in drowning is cardiac arrest due to electrolyte disturbance

D.   Postural drainage should precede BLS in near-drowning

E.   The management of near-drowning is dependent on whether it occurred in fresh or salt water

12.7 **The following are important in the correct immediate management of the near-drowning victim:**

A. Removal from the water in a vertical position

B. Maintenance of cervical spine immobilization

C. Vigorous airway suction

D. High-flow oxygen

E. Active rewarming

12.8 **The physiological effects of heat illness include:**

A. Tachycardia

B. Hypovolaemia

C. Reduced respiratory rate

D. Clotting abnormalities

E. Vasodilatation

12.9 **Features of heat illness include:**

A. Headache

B. Syncope (fainting)

C. Tachycardia

D. Hypotension

E. Muscle weakness

12.10 **The treatment of heat illness includes:**

A. Removal of the patient's clothes

B. Immersion in ice-cold water

C. Intravenous fluids

D. Blood glucose estimation

E. High-flow oxygen

12.11 **Concerning the KEMLER hazard identification system:**

A. An 'X' indicates a risk of explosion

B. A repeated number indicates an increased hazard

C. The name of the chemical is given

D. The upper number is the United Nations Product Number

E. A contact number for advice is given

SHORT NOTES

12.12 Write short notes on the different methods of heat loss.

12.13 List the methods available pre-hospital and in hospital for the rewarming of hypothermia patients.

12.14 Discuss the sources of information available at the scene of a chemical incident involving a leaking tanker.

12.15 Write short notes on the different types of radiation.

PICTURE QUIZ

12.16 What is this? How do you interpret the various sections?

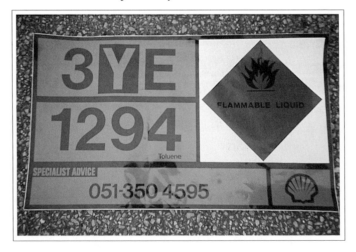

SPECIAL
INCIDENTS II

MULTIPLE CHOICE

12.1   (A) T (B) F (C) F (D) F (E) T

Severe hypothermia implies a temperature of 30°C or less. The normal body temperature is 36.5°–37.5°C. Natural wool is a good protector against heat loss.

Body temperature (°C)	Clinical features
36	Sensation of cold, stumbling, mild confusion
35	Slurred speech, incoordination, amnesia on recovery
34	Arrhythmias, typically atrial fibrillation (AF)
33	Shivering replaced by muscular rigidity
31	Pupils dilated; loss of consciousness
30	Insulin ineffective; spontaneous ventricular fibrillation (VF)
26	Major acid–base disturbance
24	Significant hypotension
23	Apnoea
18	Asystole

12.2   (A) T (B) T (C) T (D) T (E) T

Contact with dense material will increase conductive heat loss. A strong wind can significantly lower the ground temperature ('wind chill'). A child has a larger surface area:volume ratio than an adult and will lose heat at a greater rate when exposed.

12.3   (A) F (B) F (C) T (D) F (E) F

There is no evidence to show whether space blankets should be placed inside or outside a normal blanket. Space blankets protect mainly against radiant heat loss, although there is some protection against convective loss. They also reduce radiant heat absorption from the sun.

12.4   (A) F (B) T (C) F (D) T (E) T

Loss of coordination usually begins around 35°C. Shivering is lost around 33°C, when it is replaced by muscular rigidity.

12.5   2–3–4–1–5 = E

See the explanatory table in answer 12.1.

12.6   (A) F (B) T (C) F (D) F (E) F

Forty per cent of all deaths due to drowning occur in children under 5 years old. The mechanism of death in 'wet' drowning is hypoxia owing to inhaled water; in 'dry' drowning primary cardiac arrest occurs following vagal stimulation, often by the profoundly cold water. Postural drainage has no place in basic life support of the drowning victim.

12.7   (A) F (B) T (C) F (D) T (E) F

Victims of near-drowning should be removed from the water in a horizontal position and with cervical spine immobilization, where this is practical. In a vertical body, hypotension may occur as the body is lifted free from the compressive force of the water. Vigorous airway suction should be avoided: it may cause vagal stimulation or laryngeal spasm. If active rewarming is needed, this is done in hospital.

12.8   (A) T (B) T (C) F (D) T (E) T

Increasing temperature causes a rise in respiratory rate.

12.9   (A) T (B) T (C) T (D) T (E) T

These are all features of heat exhaustion.

12.10   (A) T (B) F (C) T (D) T (E) T

Immersion in cool water (not ice cold) should be considered, as this will result in rapid cooling because of the high specific heat capacity of water.

12.11   (A) F (B) T (C) F (D) F (E) F

The KEMLER-ADR system is a 40 cm × 30 cm orange board with two numbers: on top is the KEMLER code, and beneath this is the United Nations Product Number. The first KEMLER digit describes the primary hazard, and the second and third digits the secondary hazards. A repeated number signifies an intensified risk. An 'X' indicates that it must not be brought into contact with water. Unlike the UKHIS system there is no warning diamond, no action code with details of how to manage the hazard, and no manufacturer's contact number.

SHORT NOTES

12.12   The methods of heat loss are:

1. *Conduction.* This occurs through transfer of heat by direct contact with the surroundings (e.g., ground, water). It is dependent on a number of factors:

   - The greater the temperature difference between the body and the surroundings, the faster the heat is lost
   - The greater the specific heat capacity of the contact surface, the more rapidly it will take up heat
   - The surface area of contact over which heat is being lost

2. *Convection.* Air or water is warmed as it passes over the body. The rate of heat loss is not only dependent on the temperature difference of the surrounding air or water (see above, conduction), but also on the speed of movement of the air or water (i.e. the rate at which warmed air/water is replaced by fresh cold air/water).

3. *Radiation.* The body also radiates (gives off) heat to surrounding solid objects. Generally, this is much less important than conduction or convection heat loss.

4. *Evaporation.* Under normal conditions this is responsible for 20–30% of heat loss from the body, two-thirds through the skin and one-third through the respiratory tract. Evaporation of 1 g (1 ml) of water takes 0.6 kcal.

12.13 Methods available for warming the patient pre-hospital are:

1. Removal from cold environment

2. Removal of wet clothing

3. Drying body surface

4. Reduce conduction and convection losses by wrapping in multiple layers of blankets. (It is important that the patient's back is not in direct contact with a cold stretcher)

5. Warm intravenous fluids (limited availability)

6. Warm air ventilation (restricted availability, such as mountain rescue teams)

Additional methods available for warming the patient in hospital are:

1. Warm air jet duvet

2. Heat lamps

3. Rapid warm intravenous fluids where appropriate

4. Warm, humidified oxygen

5. Warm water lavage of stomach, bladder, peritoneal cavity, pleural cavity

6. Thoracic heat cradle

12.14 Sources of information at the scene of a chemical incident are:

1. *Transport emergency card (TREM card)*. This is carried in the driver's cab and will identify the load, its potential toxic effects, and will list immediate first aid (and sometimes the specific antidote).

2. *UKHIS board*. This is the board displayed on the vehicle and lists the actions by the fire service, the exact substance carried, a visible colour-coded warning and the contact telephone number of the manufacturer (see answer 12.16). The European version, the KEMLER-ADR plate, lists only the substance and the potential hazards. Either or both may be displayed on a vehicle in the UK.

3. *CHEMDATA*. This is the fire service computerized link to the National Chemical Emergency Centre at Harwell. Information is provided to the appliance at the scene via a facsimile link with fire control.

4. *National poisons unit.* In protracted incidents information may be made available at the scene by the National Poisons Information Centre at Guy's Hospital. Not only can medical advice be given, but stocks of antidote can be identified and delivery organized.

12.15   The types of radiation are:

1. α-*Radiation*. These are small, relatively heavy, positively charged particles which can travel a short distance in air (centimetres), and a very short distance through tissue (fraction of a millimetre). They are stopped by paper, clothing or a dressing.

2. β-*Radiation*. These are small, negatively charged particles. They can travel metres in air and centimetres in tissue. They are stopped by a thin sheet of aluminium or heavy clothing (military NBC clothing). β-radiation may cause skin burns.

3. γ-*Radiation and X-rays*. These travel the greatest distances in air and have the greatest tissue penetration. They are stopped by a lead shield, but the greatest protection is distance. If you double the distance, you reduce the radiation by four times (inverse square rule). Equally, if you halve the distance between you and the source, you increase your exposure by four times.

PICTURE QUIZ

12.16   This is the *United Kingdom Hazard Identification System* (UKHIS) board that is displayed on vehicles carrying hazardous substances. The components are as follows:

Emergency action code	Hazard
United Nations product number	diamond
Manufacturer's details	

The *emergency action code* tells the fire service how to fight the fire, whether to contain the chemical or wash down the drains, and what protective equipment to wear.

The *United Nations product* number is a four-digit number that relates uniquely to that chemical.

The *hazard diamond* gives a visible written and colour-coded hazard warning. The colour codes will be recognized by the fire service.

The *manufacturer's details* include a contact number for emergency advice. This is of secondary importance to informing the fire service.

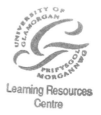

THE SICK
AND
INJURED
CHILD

Refer to Chapters 32, 33, 34, 35
and 36 of *Emergency Care:
A Textbook for Paramedics.*

MULTIPLE CHOICE

13.1 The following relate to basic life support in infants (less than 1 year):

A. Airway opening manoeuvres are identical to those for adults

B. The ratio of compression to ventilation for one rescuer is 5:1

C. Overinflation during bag-valve-mask ventilation may lead to splinting of the diaphragm

D. The compression rate is the same as for a 6-year-old

E. The hand position is one finger's breadth above the xiphisternum

13.2 The Paediatric Coma Scale:

A. Is used in head injured children up to 10 years of age

B. Has a maximum score of 12

C. Measures the best verbal, ocular and motor responses

D. Is designed to reflect the difficulty in assessing speech in children under 5 years old

E. Incorporates the Moro (startle) reflex in infants

13.3 Concerning the management of asystole in children:

A. The outcome is significantly better than in adults

B. The first dose of adrenaline is 10 μg/kg IV or ET

C. There is no role for bicarbonate

D. It is often secondary to respiratory disease

E. Drugs cannot be given through an intraosseous needle

13.4 The following formulae for children are correct:

A. Weight (kg) = [age in years + 4] × 2

B. Femoral traction (kg) = [age/2] + 2

C. Systolic BP (mmHg) = [age × 2] + 80

D. Tidal volume (ml) = 10 ml/kg

E. Fluid bolus (ml) = 50 ml/kg

13.5 Epiglottitis:

A. Is an infectious disease confined to children

B. Is usually viral

C. If considered should be confirmed by examination of the throat

D. When diagnosed should prompt an alerting message to the hospital

E. Requires the child to be transported flat with mandatory oxygen therapy

13.6 Concerning needle cricothyrotomy in children:

A. Spontaneous ventilation is possible after insertion of a 16g cannula

B. Jet insufflation is started at 1 litre/minute/year

C. Bag-valve ventilation can be adequately achieved through a 14g cannula

D. Indications for use include facial trauma

E. It will provide adequate ventilation for 15 minutes

13.7 The following are true of convulsions in children:

A. Fever is a common cause

B. Diazepam should be given during or after every convulsion

C. They may be caused by hypoglycaemia

D. Treatment with diazepam may be given IV, PR or IM

E. They increase the risk of secondary brain injury following head injury

13.8 The following are true:

A. Children are less vulnerable to injury

B. Fractured ribs are common in children

C. Small surface area renders children less vulnerable to heat loss

D. When children fall from a height they tend to land on their heads

E. Poor glycogen stores render children prone to hypoglycaemia

13.9 Concerning the paediatric airway:

A. Orotracheal intubation requires the same technique as that used for adults

B. Tidal volume of the ventilated child is best assessed by observation of the chest

C. Oropharyngeal airway size is measured by placing the airway between the angle of the jaw and the centre of the mouth

D. The tongue is relatively larger than in adults

E. The correct position of the infant's airway is with the face parallel to the hard surface on which it is lying

13.10 Paediatric normal values include:

A. Heart rate of 130 bpm in the newborn

B. Systolic blood pressure of 80 mmHg in infants

C. Circulating blood volume of 80 ml/kg in an 8-year-old

D. Respiratory rate of 20 per minute for a 10-year-old

E. Estimated weight of 20 kg for a 6-year-old

13.11 Concerning shock in children:

A. Children are better able to compensate than adults

B. Skin temperature will be affected by the ambient conditions

C. Bradycardia is a pre-terminal sign

D. Crystalloid is preferable to colloid

E. Blood pressure changes are a reliable indicator of developing shock

13.12 Relating to head injuries in children:

A. Seizures are more common than in adults

B. They are the commonest cause of death in trauma in those who reach hospital

C. Scalp laceration or haematoma may produce signs of shock

D. Diffuse cerebral oedema is the commonest pathology

E. They are more commonly associated with cervical spine injuries than in adults

SHORT ANSWERS

13.13 What modifications need to be made to the Glasgow Coma Scale when the child is less than 5 years old?

13.14 A 4-year-old pedestrian has been hit by the bumper of a car.

- What pattern of injury would you expect?
- How does this differ from the pattern in an adult?

PICTURE QUIZ

13.15 What is the cause of this rash? What are your immediate actions?

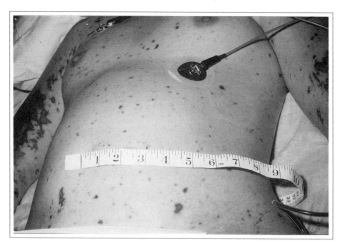

13.16 What is the diagnosis? What would you do about it?

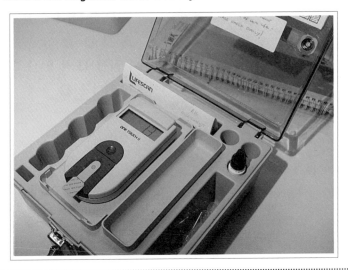

CASE HISTORY

You are called to an inner-city terraced house for a baby that has stopped breathing. On arrival you find a distraught mother in the living room with a pale, floppy baby. She says she accidentally dropped the baby off her knee 2 days ago, and that he had 'not been right' since then. The baby is breathing at about 10 per minute. You lie the baby on a table and clear its airway, then provide supplemental high-flow oxygen. The baby's breathing rate improves to 20 per minute. You decide to move rapidly to hospital. The mother does not come with you as there are three other children in the house. In the ambulance you notice that both ears are bruised, and there is a circular wound on the back of the right hand.

- What diagnosis would you consider?
- What raised your suspicion?
- What other signs might you see?

THE SICK AND INJURED CHILD

MULTIPLE CHOICE

13.1 (A) F (B) T (C) T (D) T (E) F

The airway opening manoeuvre in an infant differs from an older child or adult. As the infant has a prominent occiput, the neck is pushed into flexion in the supine position. By lifting the chin so that the face is parallel with the flat surface on which the infant is lying, the ideal airway position will be achieved. If the head is overextended, the airway will be compromised.

The ratio of compressions to ventilations for basic life support is 5:1 for all children, irrespective of whether there are one or two rescuers. The hand position for chest compressions is one finger's breadth below the inter-nipple line in infants (<1 year old), one finger's breadth above the xiphisternum in small children (1–8 years old), and two finger's breadth above the xiphisternum in older children (>8 years old).

Overinflation of the chest causes two problems. It will inflate the stomach which increases the risk of regurgitation and aspiration, and the inflated stomach will splint the diaphragm which progressively reduces the effectiveness of ventilation.

13.2 (A) F (B) F (C) T (D) T (E) F

The Paediatric Coma Scale takes account of the difficulty in assessing the verbal component of the Glasgow Coma Scale in children less than 5 years old, whose speech may be limited. The components are the same, namely the best verbal, best ocular and best motor responses, but there is a different system for scoring the verbal component. The maximum total score is 15.

The Moro reflex is a primitive startle reflex which is present in small infants (a loud noise or other stimulus causes the infant to move its arms and legs similar to a monkey trying to hold on to its mother's back).

13.3   (A) F (B) F (C) F (D) T (E) F

Cardiac arrest in children has a very poor prognosis, as it invariably follows a period of prolonged hypoxia from a respiratory illness (a primary cardiac cause such as congenital heart disaese is rare). Asystole is the commonest cardiac arrest rhythm; ventricular fibrillation is the rhythm in less than 10% of cases (compared to 90% of adults).

The first dose of adrenaline is 10 µg/kg intravenous or intraosseous, or 100 µg/kg via the endotracheal tube. All subsequent doses are 100 µg/kg.

Severe metabolic acidosis is likely, because of the prolonged hypoxia, and sodium bicarbonate has a routine role in the resuscitation of asystole in children (1 mmol/kg). A respiratory acidosis will also be present secondary to the respiratory arrest, and this is best treated by hyperventilation with 100% oxygen via an endotracheal tube.

The intraosseous route is extremely valuable in paediatric cardiac arrest. It takes approximately 10 seconds to site and, where available, it should be used as the primary venous access route for children under 6 years. The bone marrow is a central venous system and this is an additional benefit over the peripheral route.

13.4   (A) T (B) F (C) T (D) T (E) F

The formula for estimating weight is accurate from 1 to 10 years. Alternatives include asking the mother (although in the UK few mothers know the weight in kilograms), using a Broselow tape or using an Oakley Paediatric Resuscitation Chart.

The fluid bolus in children is 20 ml/kg. There is no 'rule of thumb' formula for femoral traction, which is generally not applied outside hospital as paediatric traction splints are not available to the ambulance service.

13.5   (A) F (B) F (C) F (D) T (E) F

The epiglottis is a leaf-shaped 'trap door' over the entrance to the trachea, which protects the airway during eating and drinking. Epiglottitis (inflammation of the epiglottis) is much commoner in children, but occasionally occurs in adults. It is usually bacterial, and the causative organism is *Haemophilus influenza* (serotype Pitman b). This is the organism vaccinated against by the Hib vaccine, which is now part of the routine vaccinations in children. The intention of the vaccination is to reduce the incidence of meningitis caused by the same organism, but it will be important to see if the incidence of epiglottitis is also reduced.

The throat must *not* be examined if this diagnosis is suspected, as complete airway obstruction can be precipitated. Instead, alert the hospital (as a senior anaesthetist and ear, nose and throat surgeon will be required immediately) and transport the patient in the most comfortable position. This is usually sitting up and leaning forward, perhaps on the mother's knee. Interventions are poorly tolerated: an oxygen mask can be held close to the child's face by the mother, but inserting an intravenous cannula may cause enough anxiety to again precipitate complete airway obstruction.

13.6 (A) F (B) T (C) F (D) T (E) T

Cricothyrotomy is a technique of failure, and is only considered when the airway cannot be secured by conventional means – manual manoeuvres, simple adjuncts or an endotracheal tube. The indications include upper airway obstruction from foreign body, facial trauma, burns oedema, anaphylaxis and epiglottitis. A needle cricothyrotomy is the only recommended technique for children under 12 years. If a surgical cricothyrotomy is performed in this age group (incision in the cricothyroid membrane) there is a danger that the support to the upper trachea will be lost, because the tracheal cartilage rings are immature.

The cannula must be connected to oxygen which is adjusted to 1 litre/minute/year flow rate. This is a ventilation technique so the chest should rise. If it does not, the flow rate is turned up in 1 litre/minute increments. It is a myth that a child can breathe spontaneously through a cannula, and it is a myth that effective ventilation can be provided by a resuscitation bag attached to a cannula.

This technique is a temporizing measure, and will last only 10–20 minutes. Rapid transport to hospital and an alerting message are essential.

13.7 (A) T (B) F (C) T (D) F (E) T

Fever is a common cause of convulsions in children (*febrile convulsion*). When the convulsions last less than 10 minutes, it usually indicates no serious pathology.

Every convulsion, in children or adults, does not require treatment with an anticonvulsant. A single fit that lasts less than 2 minutes would be treated by observation alone. When an anticonvulsant is required, diazepam is the usual drug that is given, rectally (5 mg in the under threes and the elderly; 10 mg in other children and adults) or intravenously (as *Diazemuls*, a less irritant suspension). It should not be given intramuscularly as its absorption is unreliable (crystallizes in muscle). Diazepam can cause respiratory depression, so be prepared to assist ventilation if required.

Following a head injury, the principal objective of management is to prevent further 'secondary' brain injury. This includes the control of any post-traumatic convulsions.

13.8 (A) F (B) F (C) F (D) T (E) T

Children are more vulnerable to injury than adults because of physical factors (less protection from elastic bony skeleton), and psychological development factors (lack of awareness of danger; inability of pedestrian to judge distance of oncoming traffic).

Fractured ribs are uncommon in children because of their elasticity, but there can be significant underlying organ injury as a result of compression.

Children have a large surface area to volume ratio and lose heat rapidly. Be aware of this and keep exposure to a minimum. A high proportion of heat is lost from the head.

When children fall they often land on their head. An analogy is if you throw a dart in the air it comes down point first, as this is the heaviest part.

Children rapidly become hypoglycaemic when stressed from injury or illness. This is because the liver glycogen stores are small, and are rapidly utilized. Do not assume that a child with a head injury is unresponsive solely from the head injury. Think hypoxia, hypovolaemia and *hypoglycaemia*.

13.9 (A) F (B) T (C) F (D) T (E) T

The infant epiglottis is relatively larger and more floppy, which necessitates the use of a straight-bladed laryngoscope and a technique where the laryngoscope blade is advanced into the oesophagus then withdrawn to pick up the epiglottis.

An oropharyngeal airway is sized in children as the vertical height between the corner of the mouth and the angle of the jaw. This is because the rounded face precludes a direct measurement of this distance.

The correct airway position in infants is with the face parallel to the firm surface on which the infant is lying (see answer to 13.1). In children over 1 year the 'adult' airway manouevre of head tilt and chin lift with the head extended can be used.

13.10   (A) T (B) T (C) F (D) T (E) T

The heart rate of a newborn baby is 120–160 per minute. The systolic blood pressure of a child is approximately twice the age in years plus 80 mmHg. The circulating blood volume at birth is about 80 ml/kg, falling to 70 ml/kg after infancy. A 1-year-old child, therefore, has only about 700 ml of blood in total (remember: weight in kilograms is estimated by [age + 4] × 2).

13.11   (A) T (B) T (C) T (D) F (E) F

Children compensate very well for shock, and maintain their systolic blood pressure. This means that blood pressure is a very poor indicator of developing shock in a child. When compensatory mechanisms fail, deterioration is usually precipitous.

Skin temperature can be a useful indicator of peripheral perfusion: a child with cold legs and a warm abdomen has a seriously compromised circulation. Of course, if the child has been exposed in a cold environment then skin temperature will be less reliable.

The pulse will rise in a linear relation to increasing blood loss until a stage of critical hypovolaemia is reached, when the pulse starts to fall again. Bradycardia in a hypovolaemic child is a pre-terminal sign. When fluid is replaced is does not matter whether the initial bolus is crystalloid (Hartman's solution) or colloid (*Haemaccel* or *Gelofusine*); the important factor is to reassess the child and repeat the bolus if the first does not significantly improve the child's clinical condition.

13.12   (A) F (B) T (C) T (D) T (E) F

Head injury is the commonest cause of death following trauma in children. The most frequently seen pathology is generalized cerebral oedema (brain swelling). Cervical spine injury is much less common in children, reflecting the elasticity of the spinal column.

In adults shock should not be attributed to a closed head injury. In small infants it is possible to lose enough blood inside an intracranial haematoma or a cephalhaematoma (a collection under the skin and galea which overly the skull) to produce signs of hypovolaemic shock.

SHORT ANSWERS

13.13 The Paediatric Coma Scale uses the same motor and ocular components as the Glasgow Coma Scale. The table below identifies the differences in the verbal component:

Glasgow Coma Scale		Paediatric Coma Scale
Orientated	5	Smiles, interacts
Confused	4	Crying (consolable)
Inappropriate	3	Crying (inconsistently consolable), moaning
Incomprehensible	2	Inconsolable, irritable
None	1	None

13.14 The pattern of injury with a child would depend on the age. A toddler will receive lower limb, pelvis, abdominal and chest injury on the same side, whereas an older child may simply receive lower limb injuries.

Additionally, a small child will be struck above his or her centre of gravity and will tend to go under the car. An older child will tend to be thrown on to the bonnet and may suffer secondary impact injuries (upper limb; head and neck).

PICTURE QUIZ

13.15 This is the characteristic rash of meningococcal septicaemia.

The immediate actions are:

- To open, clear, and secure an airway
- To give high-concentration oxygen
- To provide ventilatory support if required
- To transport rapidly to hospital and alert the Accident and Emergency Department

If a doctor is present, benzylpenicillin must be administered intramuscularly or intravenously before transport. This has been shown to improve the outcome. However, if a doctor is not present, do not delay transport waiting for one.

13.16 This picture shows a glucometer reading a low blood glucose. The normal blood glucose is 4–7 mmol/L. This is significant hypoglycaemia which requires treatment with intravenous glucose. Children respond poorly to glucagon as glycogen stores are small and are rapidly metabolized to glucose following illness or severe injury.

CASE HISTORY

The diagnosis is non-accidental injury (NAI, or child abuse). Specifically, this case is an intracerebral bleed following a severe shaking. The child was gripped by the ears during the shaking. There is also a cigarette burn to the back of the hand.

Suspicion would be raised to non-accidental injury for the following reasons:

1. *History.* The 'injury' happened several days before presentation, and does not seem consistent with the clinical findings.
2. *Signs.* A child who falls over would injure only one side of the head. Two bruised ears are not consistent with the story. Cigarette burns in this age group are unlikely to be accidental.
3. *Social circumstances.* NAI can occur in any social class, so don't prejudge!

Other features suggestive of NAI would include:

- Long bone fracture in infant too young to walk
- Multiple bruises of varying ages
- Buttock burns (from dipping in hot water)
- Lack of parental concern

THE ELDERLY PATIENT

Refer to Chapter 37 of *Emergency Care: A Textbook for Paramedics.*

MULTIPLE CHOICE

14.1 Features of depression in the elderly include:

A. Hallucinations

B. Loss of concentration

C. Hypochondriasis

D. Sleep disturbance

E. Loss of appetite

14.2 Features of the ageing psyche include:

A. Rigidity of personality

B. Increased libido

C. Bowel obsession

D. Hypochondriasis

E. Psychosis

14.3 Ocular problems in the elderly include:

A. Presbyopia

B. Glaucoma

C. Cataract

D. Macular degeneration

E. Decreased ability to judge distance

14.4   Extrinsic causes of intellectual disorder in the elderly include:

A.   Hypothyroidism

B.   Head injury

C.   Dehydration

D.   Alzheimer's disease

E.   Chronic alcohol abuse

14.5   The following are true:

A.   10% of people over 75 have some degree of hearing loss

B.   Presbyacusis is characterized by inability to hear high-pitched tones

C.   Deafness may be due to Paget's disease

D.   Paranoia may be secondary to hearing impairment

E.   Menière's disease may present with tinnitus and prostration

14.6   The following drugs commonly produce side effects in the elderly:

A.   Digoxin

B.   Paracetamol

C.   Warfarin

D.   Steroids

E.   Aspirin

14.7   The following are suggestive of the abuse of older people:

A.   Bruising on extensor surfaces

B.   Cigarette burns

C.   Laceration to the shins

D.   Head and neck bruising

E.   Stress in the carer

14.8 Features suggestive of dementia include:

A. Changes in sleep—wake pattern

B. False accusations of theft

C. Increased use of the telephone

D. Misidentification of friends or relatives

E. Increased domestic accidents

SHORT NOTES

14.9 Write short notes on the *Giants of Geriatrics*.

14.10 Discuss the methods available to you to improve communications with an elderly patient.

14.11 List the extrinsic causes of mental impairment in the elderly.

14.12 List the signs of early dementia.

PICTURE QUIZ

14.13 What potential causes of an accident can you identify in this home?

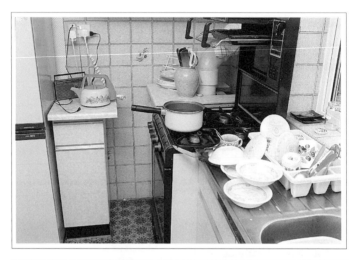

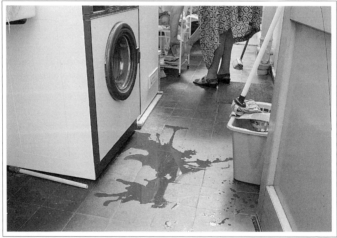

14.14 What is the diagnosis? What complications might the paramedic encounter?

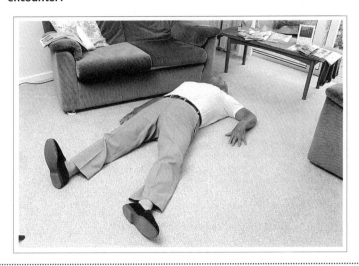

CASE HISTORY

You are called to the house of an 87-year-old whose behaviour has been causing concern to his neighbours. After much persuasion by his daughter, he agrees to be admitted to hospital.

What information might you be able to gain from:

- Talking to the patient?
- An assessment of the patient's living environment?

THE
ELDERLY
PATIENT

MULTIPLE CHOICE

14.1 (A) T (B) T (C) T (D) T (E) T

These are all features of depression in the elderly.

14.2 (A) T (B) F (C) T (D) T (E) F

Psychosis is not a feature of normal ageing.

14.3 (A) T (B) T (C) T (D) T (E) T

The four principal diseases of the ageing eye are:

- Cataract
- Macular degeneration
- Glaucoma
- Diabetic retinopathy

All of these conditions can affect acuity or clarity of vision. Poor vision will contribute to an increased likelihood of accidents. In the elderly, glaucoma can present as a unilateral headache and vomiting before visual changes become marked. Presbyopia is stiffening of the lens, which leads to a reduced ability to 'accommodate', that is to rapidly change the shape of the lens when changing from near to distant objects and vice versa. In turn, this leads to a reduced ability to judge distance, for example, the distance of moving traffic when crossing the road.

14.4 (A) T (B) T (C) T (D) F (E) T

Alzheimer's disease is a cause of *intrinsic* intellectual impairment. A full list of extrinsic causes is given in answer 14.11.

14.5 (A) F (B) T (C) T (D) T (E) T

30–40% of those over the age of 75 have some degree of hearing loss.

14.6 (A) T (B) F (C) T (D) T (E) F

Aspirin and paracetamol are usually only associated with problems if taken in deliberate overdose, which is rare in the elderly but highly significant when it does occur.

14.7 (A) F (B) T (C) F (D) T (E) T

Pretibial lacerations are common in the elderly and do not indicate abuse. Cigarette burns, on the contrary, are a feature of childhood and elderly abuse. Stress in the carer may manifest itself as abuse of the patient.

14.8 (A) T (B) T (C) T (D) T (E) T

A full list of features is given in answer 14.12.

SHORT NOTES

14.9 The Giants of Geriatrics are:

- Intellectual disorder (dementia and acute confusional states)
- Immobility, incontinence and instability (a tendency to fall)
- Visual and hearing impairment
- Depression
- Adverse drug reactions (which account for ~ 10% of acute admissions to geriatric wards)

14.10 Simple measures are most effective, such as ensuring the patient's hearing aid is switched on, or that the lighting is adequate to allow the patient to lip read.

Courtesy demands a formal introduction such as 'I am Jane Smith from the Ambulance Service' (do not be overfamiliar with the elderly, as this is often resented), and shaking hands can provide useful information about coordination, muscle strength, temperature and emotional state. When questioning an elderly person, sit at a similar level to them, speak clearly, ensure adequate lighting and do not obstruct a clear view of your mouth. Orientation may be assessed by asking the month or season: avoid patronizing questions such as 'What is the Queen's name?'

14.11 The extrinsic causes of mental impairment in the elderly are:

- Drugs
- Infection
- Hypoxia
- Dehydration
- Electrolyte and glucose disturbance
- Renal or hepatic failure
- Hypothyroidism
- Vitamin B_{12} or folate deficiency
- Head injury

14.12 Signs suggestive of early dementia are:

- Increased use of the telephone, especially during the night
- Frequent losses of key, pension book, money or jewellery
- Accusations of theft (of commonly misplaced items)
- Burning out kettles
- Leaving the gas on unlit
- Resistance to bathing and changing clothes
- Changes in sleep–wake pattern
- Soiling of clothes and neglect of personal appearance
- Leaving the house and getting lost
- Repeatedly asking the same question
- Misidentifying or failing to identify near relatives
- Speaking of the past as though it were the present, and of dead people as if they were still alive

PICTURE QUIZ

14.13 Obvious potential causes of an accident are:

- A wet floor
- Gas cooker left turned on
- Pan handle turned out

You may spot more!

14.14 The diagnosis is a fractured neck of femur. This characteristically produces a shortened, externally rotated leg.

You should first consider why the patient has fallen. There may be a medical cause for the collapse, such as a myocardial infarct, dysrhythmia, fit or hypoglycaemic episode.

Secondly, the patient may have been lying undiscovered for several hours. Hypothermia is commonly associated with this injury. Pressure sores may also be a problem.

CASE HISTORY

Information gained from talking to the patient may include:

- Current medical problems
- Past medical history
- Medications and allergies
- Social circumstances (including family and social support)

Information gained from an assessment of the patient's living environment may include:

- *The garden.* Poor maintenance may mean low interest (depression) or low ability (through disability).
- *The access.* Difficult access may be because of a fear of assault or burglary.
- *The house.* A poor state of cleanliness may be a feature of recent disability, or neglect in dementia. If the upstairs is unoccupied, it may be from poor mobility. Lack of heating may increase awareness of hypothermia.

EXTRICATION, IMMOBILIZATION AND EVACUATION

Refer to Chapters 27, 45 and 46 of
Emergency Care: A Textbook for Paramedics.

MULTIPLE CHOICE

15.1   The following statements are correct:

A   Rescue from remote places requires specialist training

B.   Entrapment relates to victims of trauma only

C.   The method of extrication should be determined by the Fire Service

D.   Immobilization of femoral shaft fractures is mandatory

E.   Paramedics are commonly part of the mountain rescue team

15.2   Snatch rescue:

A.   Includes the application of a cervical collar

B.   May be necessary before airway manoeuvres in the near-drowning casualty

C.   Is secondary to scene safety

D.   Requires two rescuers

E.   Is indicated for a seriously injured casualty in a chemical environment

15.3   Drugs commonly carried by a mountain rescue team include:

A.   Morphine

B.   Steroids

C.   Non-steroidal anti-inflammatory drugs

D.   Glucose

E.   Salbutamol

15.4   Contraindications to using a traction splint include:

A.   Ankle fractures

B.   Fracture–dislocations of the knee

C.   Pelvic fractures

D.   Fractured neck of femur

E.   Tibial shaft fracture

15.5   Manipulation of long bone fractures:

A.   Should not be undertaken pre-hospital

B.   Should include a neurovascular check before and after the procedure

C.   Requires analgesia

D.   Should be accompanied by the administration of supplementary oxygen

E.   Should not be attempted with compound fractures

15.6   Contraindications to use of the MAST suit (PASG) include:

A.   Advanced pregnancy

B.   Pelvic fractures

C.   Cardiac failure

D.   Varicose veins

E.   Ruptured diaphragm

15.7   With regard to civilian medical helicopters:

A.   They can only land at designated sites

B.   The approach is the same for all types of craft

C.   An approach can only be made with the rotors stationary

D.   Helicopters cannot fly at night

E.   Patients are at significant risk from altitude

15.8   The Kendrick Extrication Device (KED):

A.   Is an immobilization and a lifting device

B.   Provides immobilization for the cervical, thoracic and lumbar spine

C.   May cause restriction of breathing

D.   Can be used as a pelvic splint

E.   Must be removed in the resuscitation room before any X-rays are performed

....

SHORT ANSWERS

15.9   List the advantages and disadvantages of helicopter transport.

....

PICTURE QUIZ

15.10   What is this device? What are its advantages and disadvantages?

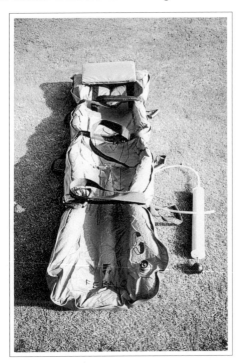

15.11 **How is the correct size chosen? Is this adequate cervical spinal immobilization?**

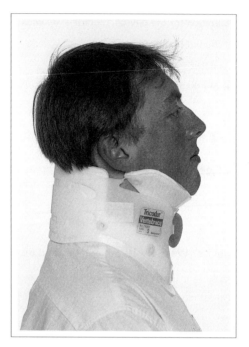

15.12 **What techniques may the Fire Service employ to improve patient access at a road traffic accident?**

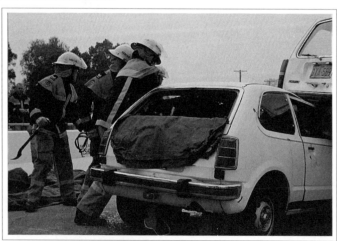

EXTRICATION, IMMOBILIZATION AND EVACUATION

MULTIPLE CHOICE

15.1 **(A)** T **(B)** F **(C)** F **(D)** F **(E)** F

Rescue from a remote place is synonymous with rescue from a *difficult* location, requiring specialist equipment and specially trained staff.

Entrapment in a vehicle may occur with a medical illness: a patient who has suffered a stroke, or a myocardial infarction is relatively entrapped, as he or she is unable to get out of the vehicle without assistance.

The ambulance officer providing the patient's care will liaise with the Fire Service, and with an immediate care doctor when present, to determine the method of extrication. In general, the ambulance officer will determine the method of extrication (for example, slide up a spinal board; lift out in a KED), but the Fire Service will determine the practicalities of how this can best be done (remove the door; remove the roof; cut the seat).

It is desirable to immobilize femoral shaft fractures to reduce pain, blood loss, prevent fat embolism and to aid packaging of the patient for transport. If there are major airway, breathing or circulation problems, these must be treated first and it may be that a continuing 'ABC' problem precludes the application of a splint.

A paramedic is not usually part of the mountain rescue team. More often the mountain rescue team will have first-aid trained member(s) and will hand over to the ambulance service at an agreed rendezvous point.

15.2   (A) F (B) T (C) T (D) F (E) T

A 'snatch rescue' is the rescue of a casualty from a hazardous and immediately life-threatening environment, such as a fire, chemical environment or near-drowning. It is often, although not exclusively, performed by the Fire Service because of the nature of the hazards. Minimal initial treatment is performed and sometimes none. There would rarely be an indication to apply a cervical collar and the complications of roughly handling a spinal injured patient will be ignored. A dead patient with or without a spinal injury is still dead.

15.3   (A) T (B) F (C) T (D) T (E) T

Essential drugs for a mountain rescue team include analgesics and drugs to treat common medical emergencies (nitrate for an angina attack; salbutamol inhaler for an asthma attack; intramuscular glucagon and oral glucose for a hypoglycaemic attack; aspirin for a myocardial infarction). Entonox is not logistical to carry, as it is too heavy, and lay members of a mountain rescue team have enjoyed the privilege of being able to administer intramuscular morphine for a number of years. This may seem odd when paramedics in the UK can at best administer a weak alternative to morphine (nalbuphine), that cannot be fully reversed by naloxone.

15.4   (A) T (B) T (C) T (D) F (E) F

A traction splint exerts traction at the ankle via some sort of hitch, and counter-traction at the pelvis. These splints are, therefore, contraindicated with ankle and *unstable* pelvic fractures (when the pelvic spring test is positive).

Traction splints are also contraindicated with a fracture–dislocation of the knee, because of the high incidence of associated vascular injury. This is particularly so with supracondylar fractures of the femur, when traction causes the fragment to tilt backwards and impinge on the vessels that run behind the knee (popliteal vessels).

A fractured neck of femur is not a contraindication. They are also of use in tibial diaphyseal fractures, particularly if associated with a femoral shaft fracture. For simple fractures of the tibia and fibula, it may be easier to apply a box splint.

15.5   (A) F (B) T (C) T (D) T (E) F

Reduction of fractures by manual traction reduces pain and blood loss, and takes the tension off essential structures, such as nerves, blood vessels, skin and muscle. Manual traction also permits the application of an appropriate splint.

Any such manipulation should include a neurovascular (nerve function and pulse) check before and after the procedure. Following the procedure the patient can be assessed as follows:

1. Nerve function*
    (a) Arm:
    - Gently wiggle fingers
    - Feel light touch on the fingers
    - Report no tingling/change of sensation
    (b) Leg:
    - Gently wiggle toes
    - Feel light touch on the toes
    - Report no tingling/change of sensation
    *(If altered before the manipulation and no change, this is acceptable but implies a high priority for evacuation)

2. Pulse
    (a) Arm:
    - Feel radial pulse
    - Normal or improved capillary return in nail bed
    - Normal or improved colour in hand
    (b) Leg:
    - Feel dorsalis pedis pulse (just outside the tendon of the big toe on the back of the foot)
    - Normal or improved capillary return in nail bed
    - Normal or improved colour in foot

Analgesia is required to effect most manipulations; with strong reassurance Entonox may be enough, but it must be administered continually for at least 2–3 minutes before the manipulation is attempted. It is important to correct the alignment of compound injuries, as well as closed fractures. Supplementary oxygen should be given to all patients with long bone fractures.

15.6 (A) T (B) F (C) T (D) F (E) T

The abdominal compartment of the MAST suit (or PASG, pneumatic anti-shock garment) should not be inflated in advanced pregnancy, or in patients with a presumed rupture of the diaphragm. Venous return to the heart is increased with a MAST suit, so contraindications also include pulmonary oedema and cardiac failure.

Varicose veins are not a contraindication. The presence of an unstable pelvic fracture is probably the only true indication that remains for this controversial device.

15.7 (A) F (B) F (C) F (D) F (E) F

The RAF publishes a manual of approved designated landing sites for helicopters carrying patients to hospital. These may be in the hospital grounds, or in a nearby school or playing field. A secondary ambulance transfer may then be required. With regards to landing at the scene, the pilot of an air ambulance helicopter may land at his or her discretion as close to the incident as is practical.

The approach to a helicopter will depend on whether it loads the patient from the side or the rear. It is usual to wait in front of the aircraft until a clear signal is given from the pilot or other crew member to approach. An approach should *never* be made from the rear when the rotors are moving: the tail rotor is difficult to see. The pilot will usually wait for all rotors to stop moving before unloading, unless the situation is critical.

The control of a helicopter during take off and landing is dependent purely on the skill of the pilot, rather than on instruments. At night, the pilot is more easily disorientated and night flying is generally avoided, unless rarely the urgency of the mission outweighs the risks. Helicopters fly at about 1000–1500 feet, and there is a minimal change in atmospheric pressure over this altitude. Problems arising on ascent and descent are, therefore, rare.

15.8 (A) T (B) T (C) T (D) T (E) F

The Kendrick Extrication Device (KED) is both an immobilization and a lifting device popular with many ambulance services. It can be left *in situ* for X-rays in the resuscitation room, although it would often be loosened and manual immobilization substituted to allow better access to the airway, and to expose the chest and abdomen for examination.

The Russel Extrication Device by comparison is only an immobilization device, and X-rays cannot be taken through it (or rather the films are unacceptable as a wire lattice is visible, superimposed on the picture).

When the chest straps are tightened there is a risk of constricting breathing, so once the patient is placed on the ambulance cot it is prudent to loosen these straps. If the splint is inverted it can be used as an improvised pelvic splint.

SHORT ANSWERS

15.9   The advantages and disadvantages of helicopter transport are:

1. *Advantages*:
   - Speed over long distance
   - Accessibility of remote places, difficult for wheeled ambulances
   - Transport of specialist medical personnel and/or equipment to the scene
   - Retrieval of the patient to a specialist trauma unit

2. *Disadvantages*:
   - High cost
   - Variable reports of overall influence on mortality and morbidity of patients within a trauma system
   - Noisy, cold, vibrating (painful fractures), nauseating and disorientating for the patient
   - Minimal pressure change effects on the patient with altitude
   - Poor patient access for interventions in flight
   - Difficult to remove a service once instituted, because of the public's perception of its value

PICTURE QUIZ

15.10   This is a vacuum mattress. A vacuum mattress is filled with miniature beads which conform rigidly to the body when the air is actively pumped out. They are light to carry, but make a poor lifting device and should be placed on top of a spinal board when carrying the patient. Smaller versions using the same principle can be used as vacuum splints for limbs, an advantage being that they will conform to the shape of a deformed limb, supporting it in the abnormal position.

15.11 A semi-rigid cervical collar is sized as follows:

- Measure the distance in 'fingers' from the base of the neck to the line of the jaw.
- Measure the same distance from the stud on the collar to the bottom of the rigid plastic (ignoring the soft foam at the bottom edge) and find the nearest approximation. Sizes (depending on the make) are a range including 'paediatric', 'short', 'regular' and 'long'.

On its own, a semi-rigid collar is *not* adequate cervical spine support. It should be accompanied by continuing manual immobilization until this is replaced by sandbags + tape, or a headbox.

15.12 Improved patient access can be afforded by a number of techniques including:

- Opening a jammed door, or breaking a window
- Removing a door
- Removing the windscreen (on its own if non-bonded)
- Removing the roof, or folding back the roof
- Removing another patient
- Removing the steering wheel
- Pulling forward the dashboard, when intruding

PREGNANCY, CHILDBIRTH AND THE NEONATE

Refer to Chapters 47, 48, 49 and 50 of *Emergency Care: A Textbook for Paramedics.*

MULTIPLE CHOICE

16.1   The following are true in pregnancy:

A.   There is an increased risk of regurgitation and aspiration

B.   The tongue becomes relatively larger

C.   Intubation is made more difficult by engorged breasts

D.   Cricothyrotomy is made more difficult by neck obesity

E.   The trachea elongates with associated chest wall changes

16.2   Changes in breathing in pregnancy include:

A.   Splinting of the diaphragm

B.   Decreased tidal volume

C.   Increased respiratory rate

D.   Increased oxygen carrying capacity

E.   Splaying of the ribs

16.3   Circulatory changes in pregnancy include:

A.   An increase in the blood volume by 50%

B.   A normal increase in systolic blood pressure by up to 30 mmHg

C.   Hypotension in the supine position

D.   ST segment elevation on the ECG

E.   A normal increase in the heart rate by 5–10 beats per minute

16.4 The following are true in labour:

A. The second stage of labour lasts about 5–20 minutes

B. 'Labour' starts after the waters have broken

C. The second stage of labour refers to the time from crowning to delivery of the baby

D. Syntometrine is given with the delivery of the anterior shoulder

E. The cord must be divided between two clamps

16.5 Concerning the stages of labour:

A. The first stage ends when the cervix is 10 cm dilated

B. The fetal head is visible at the introitus at the end of the first stage

C. During the second stage the fetal heart rate normally drops to around 100 per minute

D. The placenta is delivered by gentle traction

E. Placental expulsion may be stimulated by placing the baby on the breast

16.6 Common associations with ectopic pregnancy are:

A. Shoulder tip pain

B. Onset between 5 and 12 weeks of pregnancy

C. Heavy vaginal bleeding

D. Lower abdominal pain on one side

E. Hypovolaemic shock

16.7 The following features are characteristic of placental abruption:

A. The placental position is usually abnormal

B. The fetus is often compromised

C. There is often little or no vaginal bleeding

D. The diagnosis is suggested by abdominal pain

E. It follows abdominal trauma

16.8   Eclampsia:

A.   May present with fitting

B.   Is preceded by hypertension and protein in the urine

C.   Will improve with delivery of the baby

D.   Is associated with a high fetal mortality

E.   Is associated with peripheral oedema in the mother

16.9   With trauma in pregnancy:

A.   Maternal hypotension is a late feature

B.   Caval compression must be relieved with a pelvic wedge

C.   The priority with abdominal trauma after 35 weeks is to deliver the baby

D.   Uterine haemorrhage may be concealed

E.   Uterine rupture is suggested by severe pain and a fetus that is easy to feel

16.10   Concerning neonatal resuscitation:

A.   The safety valve on a neonatal bag-valve mask is set to 50 cmH$_2$O

B.   The correct endotracheal tube size for the newborn is 2.5–3.5 mm internal diameter

C.   Opiates given to the mother can cause respiratory depression in the baby

D.   The circulating blood volume in a neonate is $\sim$500 ml

E.   Cold stress may result in hypoglycaemia

SHORT ANSWERS

16.11   Discuss your actions on discovering a prolapsed cord.

16.12   What are the causes of antepartum haemorrhage (APH)? How would you treat an APH?

PICTURE QUIZ

16.13 What would you do?

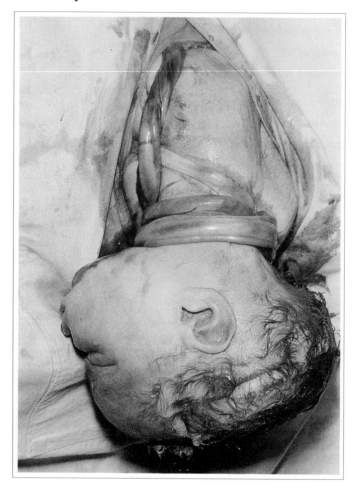

16.14 What is this called? What would you do?

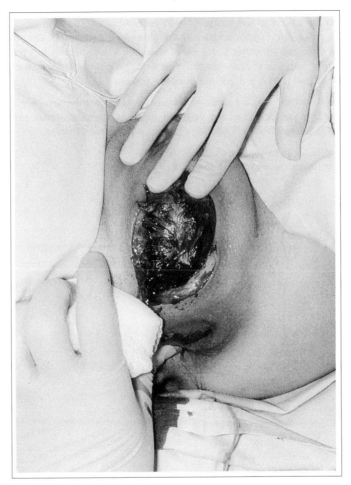

CASE HISTORY

You are called to the house of a 14-year-old girl by her mother, who dials 999 when she cannot rouse her daughter in the morning. On arrival she can give you no other story other than the daughter has put on a lot of weight in the last few months. You find the girl unresponsive and fitting in her bed. What are your immediate actions?

The fits stop after a couple of minutes and before departure you notice that she has facial and leg swelling, and has a gravid uterus extending above the umbilicus. The blood pressure is 225/145 mmHg.

- What is the diagnosis?
- What other treatment does she require?

PREGNANCY, CHILDBIRTH AND THE NEONATE

MULTIPLE CHOICE

16.1   (A) T (B) F (C) T (D) T (E) F

In pregnancy there is relaxation of the gastro-oesophageal junction with an increased risk of regurgitation and aspiration. This is particularly important in illness or injury when a reduced level of response further increases the risk to the airway. Aspiration pneumonitis when it occurs (Mendelssohn's syndrome) has a poor prognosis.

Intubation is made more difficult in advanced pregnancy because of an obese neck; additionally, the engorged breasts may make manipulation of the laryngoscope handle into the mouth difficult. Cricothyrotomy may also be more difficult when the neck is more obese.

16.2   (A) T (B) F (C) F (D) F (E) T

The tidal volume (volume of air exchanged with each breath) is increased by 40% in pregnancy. The diaphragm is elevated by the gravid uterus, and there is a reduction in the residual volume (volume of air left in the lungs on expiration) of the lungs. The respiratory rate is unchanged in pregnancy.

There is a 'physiological' anaemia in pregnancy because of a greater increase in plasma volume relative to the increase in red cell mass. This probably optimizes the blood flow through the placental bed and, therefore, materno-fetal oxygen exchange. However, the oxygen-carrying capacity per unit of blood is reduced because of the anaemia.

16.3   (A) T (B) F (C) T (D) F (E) T

The blood volume increases by 50% in the second trimester (middle 12 weeks) of pregnancy, and the cardiac output increases by 1–1.5 L/min. The heart rate may increase by 5–10 beats per minute to an average of 85–90 per minute.

Systolic blood pressure consistently falls in the second trimester by 5–15 mmHg. Any rise in blood pressure should be regarded seriously and may indicate pre-eclampsia (see answer 16.8). Hypotension in the supine position is caused by inferior vena caval compression from the gravid uterus (main venous return from the legs is compressed by the uterus).

ECG changes in pregnancy include flattened or inverted T-waves in leads III and AVF, and atrial ectopics.

16.4   (A) F (B) F (C) F (D) T (E) T

Labour (from the Latin *laboro*, I work) is the act of propulsion of the fetus and placenta from the uterus. It starts with the onset of contractions, not the waters breaking as this can be delayed.

Stage I is from onset of contractions to full dilatation of the cervix. It lasts 12 hours on average.

Stage II is from full dilatation to complete expulsion of the baby. It lasts one hour on average.

Stage III is the expulsion of the placenta. It normally lasts from 5–20 minutes.

The cord should be divided between two clamps, otherwise there is the danger of neonatal or maternal haemorrhage from the unclamped end of the cord.

Syntometrine 0.5 mg is an oxytocic drug (stimulates contractions) and is given to reduce the chance of post-partum haemorrhage (bleeding from the uterus after delivery of the baby).

16.5   (A) T (B) F (C) F (D) T (E) T

The normal fetal heart rate is 120–160 beats per minute (usually 135–150). Bradycardia or tachycardia is a sign of fetal hypoxia.

The placenta is delivered by gentle traction, with counter traction on the abdomen to prevent the uterus from inverting. The placenta should be checked to ensure that all the cotelydons ('leaves') are present (if retained in the uterus, the uterus cannot fully contract and there is a risk of post-partum haemorrhage).

Placental expulsion may be stimulated by placing the baby on the breast which stimulates the release of naturally occurring oxytocin.

16.6   (A) T (B) T (C) F (D) T (E) T

An ectopic pregnancy is a pregnancy that occurs outside the cavity of the uterus. The incidence in the United Kingdom is ~1:300 pregnancies, and virtually all occur in the Fallopian tubes (the tubes connecting the ovaries to the uterus).

The ectopic pregnancy manifests at 5–12 weeks after conception, and amenorrhoea (absent period) may not have been noticed. Pain is in the lower abdomen, initially to one side. Bleeding is usually mild. The abdomen may be rigid when there is rupture of the tube and bleeding into the abdomen. Shoulder pain occurs when the blood tracks up the gutters either side of the spine and irritates the diaphragm, which shares the same sensory innervation as the shoulder.

This is a gynaecological emergency and the hypovolaemia can be life-threatening.

16.7   (A) F (B) T (C) T (D) T (E) T

Placental abruption is bleeding from the bed of a normally sited placenta in the upper part (upper segment) of the uterus. An abnormally sited placenta in the lower segment is termed placenta praevia.

Vaginal bleeding may be absent ('concealed') or revealed. Often there is little bleeding, and shock is disproportionate to the show. Pain is severe.

The causes and associations of placental abruption include trauma, pre-eclampsia, multiparity (multiple previous pregnancies) and previous abruption.

16.8   (A) T (B) T (C) T (D) T (E) T

Pre-eclampsia is a rise in blood pressure in the final 12 weeks of pregnancy, associated with proteinuria and oedema. The incidence in the UK is about 10–15% of pregnancies. It nearly always precedes eclampsia.

Impending eclampsia is heralded by headache and blurred vision (from rising intracranial pressure), epigastric pain (from liver oedema), a falling urinary output and a rapidly rising blood pressure.

Eclampsia presents with fitting and coma. There is a high fetal mortality. The majority of cases start in pregnancy (60%) and are improved by delivery; 20% occur during delivery, and 20% occur after delivery.

16.9 (A) T (B) T (C) F (D) T (E) T

As the maternal blood volume is increased by up to 50%, hypotension is a late sign after blood loss in trauma.

Caval compression in the supine position can seriously impair venous return to the heart and a wedge (a pillow, or rolled jacket) should be placed under the right hip *even when spinal injury has not been excluded*.

The priority in resuscitation is the mother. *Look after the mother and the fetus will look after itself.*

16.10 (A) F (B) T (C) T (D) F (E) T

The safety valve on a neonatal bag-valve-mask apparatus is set to 30 cmH$_2$O pressure in order to reduce the risk of pulmonary barotrauma (a pneumothorax induced by high inflation pressure).

The average endotracheal tube size for a full-term newborn baby is 3.0 mm internal diameter, but it is sensible to have the half-size above and below available.

Opiates given to the mother are well recognized to cause repiratory depression in the infant. In this case the airway and ventilation of the baby are supported, and intramuscular naloxone should be administered.

The circulating blood volume of a baby is 80 ml/kg. A full-term baby weighs approximately 3 kg, so the estimated blood volume is 240 ml.

Cold stress may result in hypoglycaemia, increased oxygen consumption, hypoxia and acidosis. It must be avoided by drying the baby and wrapping in a (preferably warm) towel.

SHORT ANSWERS

16.11 A prolapsed cord occurs when the membranes rupture and the presenting part (usually the head) is poorly fitting in the pelvis. A poorly fitting presenting part may be a result of prematurity, a small baby, or a multiple pregnancy.

If immediate delivery is imminent, then assist the delivery. If delivery is not imminent, keep the cord warm and moist, with minimal handling. If you touch the cord too frequently or handle it roughly you may cause cord spasm (with resultant fetal hypoxia). Turn the mother into the lateral position and raise the hips up on one or two pillows. Do not try to replace the cord above the presenting part, as this not only induces spasm but further loops of cord may fall down.

16.12 Antepartum haemorrhage is vaginal bleeding after 28 weeks gestation, but before the onset of labour. The causes are:

Placental abruption	50%
Placenta previa	20%
Cervix/vagina pathology	4%
Blood disorder	1%
No cause found	25%

Placental abruption is described in answer 16.7. Placenta praevia is when the placenta lies abnormally in the lower segment, over the cervical os. Bleeding may occur before labour, or when the cervix starts to dilate in the first stage of labour. If placenta praevia is suspected, *a vaginal examination must **not** be performed.*

The action is to secure the airway and support ventilation where required. High concentration oxygen should be given. Intravenous access and fluids will be started depending on the transit time to hospital. This is an obstetric emergency and the hospital should be given an alerting message.

PICTURE QUIZ

16.13 This is a cord around the neck. If not treated immediately the baby will die. A manipulation of the cord may be attempted, but if this fails, clamp the cord in two places and divide it with scissors.

16.14 This is crowning of the baby's head. The baby is about to deliver. Apply gentle pressure on the vertex to control the head. Suck out the nose and mouth with a neonatal aspirator when the face appears. Assist the delivery of the baby.

CASE HISTORY

The immediate actions for any patient who is fitting are to clear and secure the airway. Use suction to clear the airway, and insert a nasopharyngeal airway adjunct. It is difficult to assist ventilation in the tonic or clonic phases of a fit, but should the fit resolve spontaneously, assisted ventilation is provided if necessary. High-concentration oxygen should be given whether spontaneously ventilating or with assisted ventilation. If the convulsion continues, give diazepam 10 mg per rectum.

The diagnosis in this case is eclampsia. As the mother is unaware of the pregnancy, it seems to have been concealed by the daughter. This means that the warning signs of pre-eclampsia (hypertension, proteinuria, and oedema) that would have been discovered in an antenatal clinic have been missed.

The patient requires rapid transport to hospital for an emergency delivery of the baby.

PSYCHIATRY AND SUBSTANCE ABUSE

Refer to Chapters 51, 52, 53 and 54 of *Emergency Care: A Textbook for Paramedics.*

MULTIPLE CHOICE

17.1   Features of the alcohol dependence syndrome include:

A.   Drinking a wide range of alcoholic drinks

B.   Increased alcohol tolerance

C.   Replacement of normal activities by drinking

D.   Early morning drinking

E.   Delirium tremens

17.2   Physical consequences of alcohol abuse include:

A.   Heart failure

B.   Hypoglycaemia

C.   Acute onset palsy of eye muscles

D.   Muscle weakness

E.   Increased incidence of falls

17.3   Features of alcohol withdrawal include:

A.   Desperate craving for alcohol

B.   Confusion

C.   Convulsions

D.   Hallucinations

E.   High breath and blood alcohol levels

17.4 Features of opiate overdose include:

A. Coma

B. Convulsions

C. Hyperventilation

D. Dilated pupils

E. Full reversibility with naloxone

17.5 Symptoms commonly associated with LSD (speed) include:

A. Sense of despair

B. Coma

C. Constricted pupils

D. Pyrexia

E. Hypotension

17.6 Amphetamines:

A. Are safe recreational drugs

B. Are sold on the streets as 'acid'

C. May produce a schizophrenia-like psychosis

D. Are hallucinogenic drugs

E. Cause depression

17.7 Ecstasy:

A. Is associated with pyrexia and heat exhaustion

B. Deaths are related to more than 10 g of the drug being ingested

C. May cause death by cardiac dysrhythmia

D. Is known on the street as 'Special K'

E. Has a strong association with cerebrovascular accident

17.8   Concerning the abuse of volatile substances:

A.   Mouth-to-mouth ventilation is contraindicated

B.   Perforation of the nasal septum may occur

C.   Death is often from cardiac dysrhythmias

D.   Death is often from asphyxia

E.   The toxic substances include toluene

17.9   Features of acute mania include:

A.   Suicidal ideation

B.   Flight of ideas

C.   Paranoia

D.   Indiscreet behaviour

E.   Rapid speech

17.10   The following are true of a psychotic patient:

A.   The patient may be detained against his or her will for assessment and treatment

B.   Schizophrenia produces hallucinations and thoughts of external control

C.   Patients may be physically restrained

D.   The police may detain the patient under Section 136

E.   Air ambulance transport is contraindicated

17.11   Features of post-traumatic stress disorder include:

A.   Poor sleep

B.   Flashbacks to the incident

C.   Poor concentration at work

D.   Marital disharmony

E.   Hallucinations

SHORT ANSWERS

17.12   Discuss the strategies for dealing with a violent patient.

17.13   What is critical incident stress debriefing? When should it be undertaken, and by whom?

PICTURE QUIZ

17.14 What would you do?

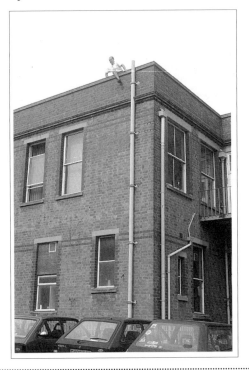

CASE HISTORY

You are called to the house of a 40-year-old widow by a concerned neighbour. You see through the living room window that she has slashed her wrists and is lying on the floor in a pool of blood.

- What action would you take?
- What are your options if she refuses treatment?

PSYCHIATRY AND SUBSTANCE ABUSE

MULTIPLE CHOICE

17.1   (A) T (B) T (C) T (D) T (E) T

An alcohol-dependent patient will often use a wide range of alcoholic drinks, being more concerned about quantity than quality. Liver enzymes will be induced and a tolerance to alcohol develops, so that more needs to be consumed for the same effect. Early morning drinking to avoid withdrawal symptoms is seen, but if there is abstension (whether deliberate, or accidental following a hospital admission), then an acute confusional state may develop – *delirium tremens*, or 'DTs'.

Other features of this syndrome are social and psychological:

1. *Social*
   - Marital disharmony/wife-beating
   - Sickness from work
   - Increased risk of accidents (road; industry)
   - Increased crime
   - Vagrancy

2. *Psychological*
   - Increased suicide
   - Sexual problems

17.2   (A) T (B) T (C) T (D) T (E) T

The physical consequences of alcohol abuse are protean and virtually every body system can be adversely affected. Heart failure may occur because of cardiomyopathy, but this is rare. Hypoglycaemia is seen because poor diet and liver damage (fatty change; alcoholic hepatitis or cirrhosis) result in poor glycogen stores.

Ocular palsy occurs in *Wernicke's encephalopathy* as a result of degenerative changes in the brainstem and thalamus attributable to thiamine (vitamin B_1) deficiency. A staggering gait and confusion are also seen.

Muscle weakness occurs as a result of a myopathy, which may contribute to the increased incidence of falls.

17.3 (A) T (B) T (C) T (D) T (E) F

The spectrum of alcohol withdrawal symptoms is wide. Moderate symptoms would include tremor, nausea and retching, sweating, mood swings and muscle cramps. More severe symptoms would include hallucinations and convulsions.

Delirium tremens occurs 2–4 days after alcohol withdrawal and is a combination of vivid hallucinations (visual and auditory), delusions (irrational beliefs), confusion and agitation. DTs are also associated with convulsions and Wernicke's encephalopathy (see answer 17.2). Most patients have existing liver damage. DTs may be precipitated by trauma or infection.

17.4 (A) T (B) F (C) F (D) F (E) T

Opiate overdose will cause coma. The clues to the aetiology are pinpoint pupils and needle track marks. The immediate cause of death is usually respiratory depression (hypoventilation). Hypotension also occurs. The effects of the overdose can be reversed by naloxone, but in an addict this may precipitate acute withdrawal symptoms and produce an aggressive patient. The half-life of naloxone is short, and toxic effects of the overdose may reappear requiring a further dose of naloxone.*

Opiate *withdrawal* effects include agitation, sweating, tachycardia, dilated pupils and abdominal cramps. 'Goose flesh' is characteristically described. Convulsions may occur.

*Naloxone will fully reverse the effects of morphine or diamorphine (heroin, smack), but not nalbuphine or buprenorphine

17.5 (A) T (B) F (C) F (D) T (E) F

Lysergic acid diethylamide (LSD, 'speed' or 'whizz') is a hallucinogenic drug. It is available in tablet or stamp (impregnated paper logo) form. A tiny dose (1 μg) is required to produce an effect after about 30 minutes.

Users note changes in perception of time, colour, sound and surroundings which last up to 12 hours. Judgement may be affected. Trying to fly is a well-recognized response which is invariably unsuccessful!

A sense of despair occurs on a 'bad trip' and may be associated with acute depression.

Physiological effects include dilated pupils, tachycardia, hypertension and pyrexia.

17.6 (A) F (B) T (C) T (D) T (E) T

Amphetamines are a stimulant ('upper') drug, which can be abused orally, intravenously or subcutaneously.

Characteristically they produce excitement, euphoria and an increased capacity for concentration or physical activity. Physiological effects include dilated pupils and tachycardia. As the drug wears off there may be fatigue, headache and depression.

With chronic abuse, a schizophrenia-like psychosis may occur, with paranoid ideas and hallucinations as prominent features.

17.7 (A) T (B) F (C) T (D) F (E) F

Ecstasy (or 'E') is *3,4-methylene dioxymethamphetamine* (MDMA). It is an increasingly common drug of misuse amongst the young adult population, being particularly associated with 'raves'.

Adverse effects are associated with dehydration, pyrexia and a heat exhaustion picture. Death may follow cardiac dysrhythmias. Treatment should be directed towards rehydration, cooling and support of ABCs.

More than 10 g of paracetamol (20 tablets) is a potentially lethal dose. One ecstasy tablet may be lethal. Ketamine is known on the streets as 'Special K'.

17.8 (A) F (B) T (C) T (D) F (E) T

'Glue sniffing' or the abuse of other volatile substances is popular amongst the older child population. With chronic use, nasal septal ulceration and perforation may occur.

The effects of inhaling the volatile substances include cardiac dysrhythmias and convulsions. Mouth-to-mouth ventilation is not contraindicated, but an airway adjunct (such as a pocket mask) is always preferred aesthetically.

17.9 (A) F (B) T (C) F (D) T (E) T

Mania and depression are opposites of mood, and a 'manic–depressive' will swing between these extremes. The depressive will be slow of thought, feel worthless and may consider suicide. The manic individual will have rapid thought ('flight of ideas', changing from one topic to another mid-sentence), rapid speech and an inflated self-image. Activity is generally increased at work, physically and socially. Attention from the emergency services may be drawn by indiscreet behaviour or performance of risky pursuits.

17.10   (A) T (B) T (C) T (D) T (E) T

A psychotic patient may be detained against their will for assessment and treatment under the Mental Health Act, if it is considered they are in danger of harming themself or others. The police may remove an individual to a 'place of safety' under Section 136, whom they consider in danger of harming himself or herself, or others. An Accident and Emergency department is *not* a place of safety. It is still considered to be a public place. A place of safety would be the secure wing of a psychiatric unit.

In schizophrenia, the patient may describe thought insertion, and may feel that he or she is being controlled externally.

Physical restraint is a difficult issue. In the United States the hospital is negligent if a patient causes himself or herself further harm while in the care of the hospital, so the threshold to restrain is low, and restraint is effected by straps on to the bed or trolley. In the UK it would be reasonable to restrain a patient to prevent further harm, but this rarely involves anything other than manual restraint pre-hospital or in an Accident and Emergency Department.

Air ambulance transport is contraindicated because of the unpredictability of the patient, who may jeopardize other passengers and crew.

17.11   (A) T (B) T (C) T (D) T (E) F

Post-traumatic stress disorder is often referred to in the context of a major incident, but equally may occur after a single casualty incident. It may affect the patients, relatives and carers alike. Symptoms can be delayed in onset for many months.

Critical incident stress debriefing by ambulance colleagues, formal counselling by professional counsellors and even psychiatric assistance can be required.

SHORT ANSWERS

17.12   The strategies for dealing with a violent patient include:

1. *Avoiding the situation.* Do not place yourself at unnecessary risk. Summon the assistance of the police if required.
2. *Defusing the situation.* Take a non-aggressive stance, for example, sit down if the patient is standing. Do not use aggressive body language such as finger pointing. Speak calmly and do not try to antagonize.

3. *Restraining the patient.* This is less satisfactory and is best done with the assistance of the police. Remember, however, that a patient may be confused and aggressive because of hypoxia, and it may be in the patient's interests to be restrained to seek urgent hospital treatment.

17.13 Critical incident stress debriefing occurs at several levels. Informally this is the debriefing of the two members of the ambulance crew at the ambulance station over a cup of tea, perhaps involving the opinions of their peers. Hopefully, there will also be some immediate feedback from Accident and Emergency clinicians when a difficult case is brought into the hospital.

At a slightly higher level there may be more formal debriefing by the station officer or local training officer. Individuals should feel that they can speak openly, and should be asked what went well and what could have been done differently. This will allow reflection over the incident and an opportunity to consolidate positive messages and to learn from mistakes.

After a major incident it is likely that the critical incident stress debriefing will be led by a counsellor or clinical psychologist. Persons having difficulty with coping with the incident will be identified and offered further counselling, and a small number may require formal psychiatric assistance.

PICTURE QUIZ

17.14 There is no textbook answer to this situation. Your objectives, should you be first on the scene, are to calm the patient, to establish a rapport, to keep the patient talking so as to distract from the suicidal intent, and if possible to 'talk them down'. This role of counsellor will often be taken by the police, who may employ a professional for exactly this purpose. Clearly, if the patient does jump it becomes an ambulance responsibility to assess and treat the injured, or to declare that resuscitation is inappropriate.

CASE HISTORY

Access must be gained to the house. This would usually be a police responsibility. Once inside ensure the scene is made safe, and the knife is removed from harm's way. Protect yourself with gloves before offering treatment. Reassure the patient, and assess and treat along ABC lines. Most bleeding will stop with direct pressure and elevation. Be alert to symptoms of tingling, numbness or loss of function that may indicate associated nerve or tendon injury.

In general, a person who refuses treatment cannot be forced into an ambulance and taken to hospital. If it is considered that the patient is at continued risk of taking their own life (and this assumption would have to be made by the ambulance crew) then either:

- Contact Ambulance Control to arrange for the general practitioner to attend for an assessment to be made as to whether the patient should be detained in hospital under the Mental Health Act
- Allow the police to transport the patient to a 'place of safety' (this does not include an Accident and Emergency department)

If the patient is so ill that emergency life-saving treatment is required then common lore allows the ambulance service (and the hospital clinicians) to provide this treatment against the wishes of the patient, in their own best interests.

MAJOR INCIDENTS

Refer to Chapters 55 and 56 of *Emergency Care: A Textbook for Paramedics.*

MULTIPLE CHOICE

18.1   In Health Service terms, the following are important in determining whether an incident is a 'major incident':

A.   The number of casualties

B.   The severity of casualties

C.   The type of injuries

D.   The number of dead

E.   The location of the incident

18.2   The following are key ambulance service appointments at a major incident:

A.   Primary Triage Officer

B.   Ambulance Loading Officer

C.   Ambulance Parking Officer

D.   Mortuary Officer

E.   Ambulance Safety Officer

18.3   The following are true of personal equipment at a major incident:

A.   A hospital Mobile Medical Team may be refused admission to the scene if its members are inappropriately dressed

B.   All the Incident Officers will wear a blue and white chequered tabard

C.   Doctors will wear white hats with green lettering

D.   Ear protection should be carried

E.   Medical teams will wear red clothing in Scotland

18.4   Concerning scene command and control:

A.   The Fire Service will control the operational area in the presence of fire or chemical hazard

B.   The Police are in overall control at the scene

C.   The Medical Incident Officer has overall responsibility for medical and ambulance resources

D.   The operational or bronze control refers to the Incident Officers at the scene

E.   There is always a gold medical commander

18.5   Concerning the dead at the scene:

A.   The dead are held at the scene in a temporary mortuary

B.   The triage colour for the dead is blue

C.   The dead should not be moved until they have been photographed

D.   The dead are the responsibility of the Coroner

E.   The ambulance service are responsible for removing the dead from the scene

18.6   The following are acceptable key words over the radio:

A.   Roger

B.   Over and out

C.   10-4

D.   Say again

E.   Acknowledge

18.7   Methods of communication at a major incident include:

A.   Pager

B.   Field telephone

C.   UHF radio

D.   Whistle

E.   Hand signals

18.8   Disadvantages of a mobile telephone at the scene are:

A.   Limited cellular capacity may be completely swamped

B.   Loss of coordination of information

C.   Geographical blackspots

D.   Interference with medical monitoring equipment

E.   Less talk time than a radio

18.9   The following relate to triage:

A.   It is performed once only

B.   It literally means 'to divide into three'

C.   It assigns a priority for treatment or evacuation

D.   The expectant category are those who cannot be treated at the scene

E.   A red category means 'urgent' treatment is required

18.10   Concerning Mobile Medical Team equipment:

A.   It must complement rather than duplicate ambulance service equipment

B.   It should be held at an equipment dump adjacent to the Casualty Clearing Station

C.   Amputation equipment should be carried by each team

D.   Resupply will routinely be from the parent hospital

E.   It should reflect that most treatment at the scene is directed towards the 'ABCs'.

SHORT ANSWERS

18.11   List the functions of the police at the scene of a major incident.

18.12   What is the phonetic spelling of the following drugs?

- Entonox
- Morphine
- Ketamine

18.13   Draw how you would optimally organize a Casualty Clearing Station.

18.14   What is the difference between the *triage sieve* and the *triage sort*?

PICTURE QUIZ

18.15 You are the first ambulance crew to arrive. What are your priorities?

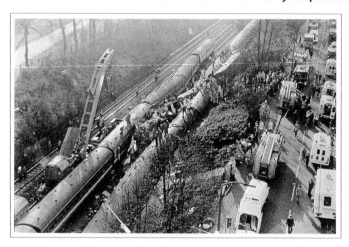

18.16 What are the triage priorities commonly used at a major incident? How is the expectant category represented on a triage label?

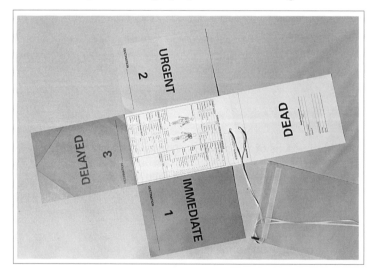

CASE HISTORY

You are appointed as the Triage Officer and encounter the following casualties at the scene. Assign a colour-coded priority to each of them.

1. A 20-year-old woman. She runs towards you screaming hysterically. She has multiple facial, chest and arm lacerations.
2. An elderly man with a right lower leg traumatic amputation. He is not breathing, and there is no palpable pulse.
3. A young boy with an open head injury and visible brain. He is unresponsive to pain and breathing at 4 per minute. He has a very thready and rapid carotid pulse.
4. A middle-aged woman with a closed fracture of the right femur and Colles' fracture of the right. She is alert, but in considerable pain. Her respiratory rate is 25 per minute and pulse 125 per minute.

MAJOR
INCIDENTS

MULTIPLE CHOICE

18.1   (A) T (B) T (C) T (D) F (E) T

A major incident in Health Service terms is any incident where the
number, severity or type of live casualties, or by its location, requires
extraordinary arrangements by the health services.

18.2   (A) T (B) T (C) T (D) F (E) T

The *Primary Triage Officer* performs triage where the patient is first found;
secondary triage occurs at the Casualty Clearing Station. The *Ambulance
Loading Officer* will determine the order of evacuation of casualties, their
destination and the mode of transport. The *Ambulance Parking Officer* will
marshall ambulance vehicles as they arrive at the scene and, through
liaison with the Loading Officer, establish a flow of vehicles forward to the
Casualty Clearing Station. The *Ambulance Safety Officer* is appointed to
ensure all health service personnel are appropriately dressed, and that all
hazards to health service personnel are identified. The police are in
charge of the body holding area (see below), and there would be no
requirement for a mortuary officer from the ambulance service.

18.3   (A) T (B) F (C) F (D) T (E) T

The Ambulance Safety Officer will refuse admission to the scene of health
services personnel who are inappropriately dressed. The *Police* Incident
Officer wears a blue and white chequered tabard, the Fire Incident
Officer wears red and white, and the Ambulance Incident Officer wears
green and white. Doctors and nurses will wear green helmets with white
lettering (white with green lettering is worn by the Ambulance Service).
In Scotland, medical teams currently wear red overalls and red helmets.

18.4   (A) T (B) T (C) F (D) F (E) F

Command operates vertically, within each emergency service; control operates across the services. The police are in overall control at the scene ('tactical', or 'silver' level control), but the fire service will be in control of the immediately hazardous area ('operational', or 'bronze' control). The Medical Incident Officer is responsible for all medical and nursing assets at the scene, but the Ambulance Incident Officer is responsible for all ambulance assets. The operational (bronze) command, therefore, refers to the Forward Incident Officers. The Incident Officers represent tactical (silver) command. A 'gold' (strategic) medical commander is usually *not* appointed.

18.5   (A) F (B) F (C) T (D) T (E) F

The dead are held at the scene in a body holding area. The temporary mortuary is the place where the pathological examinations will take place. The triage colour for the dead is black or white, depending on the labelling system used. Ideally the dead should not be moved until they have been photographed, as they are part of the forensic evidence. The dead may be moved earlier to gain access to the living, or to protect a body or body part from destruction by fire or chemical. The dead are the responsibility of the Coroner, or Procurator Fiscal in Scotland, and it is a police responsibility to organize the removal of the dead from the scene.

18.6   (A) T (B) F (C) F (D) T (E) T

'Roger' is equivalent to 'OK'. Each radio message is either suffixed 'over' (the other party is to speak) or 'out' (no response is required, the message is ended). 'Acknowledge' requires the receiver to *say back* the important part of the message to ensure it has been understood.

18.7   (A) T (B) T (C) T (D) T (E) T

The radio is very busy in a major incident, and alternative forms of communication should be considered. A message pager can be used to send an individual or group messages. A field telephone system may be set up rapidly to communicate from a number of fixed points around the scene, and such a system would be available by request from British Telecom. Whistle blasts to the fire service mean evacuate the area. If a whistle is used, predetermined signals should be agreed. Similarly, hand signals are commonly used in the military to communicate across open ground, but in civilian practice the signals must be agreed in advance.

18.8 (A) T (B) T (C) T (D) F (E) F

There are two principal disadvantages of a cellular telephone: loss of coordination, and overloading of the system. Coordination is lost when messages are passed by telephone which are not logged centrally. Overload is more common with the analogue system than with the digital network, which has about four times the number of available cells. Phones may be modified to operate on a restricted number of cells following Cabinet Office approval, and this system is known as ACCOLC (Access Overload Control). ACCOLC may be instituted by the police when the cellular system is overcrowded.

18.9 (A) F (B) F (C) T (D) F (E) F

Triage means to sift or to sort, and it is only coincidence that there are three main triage categories. It is a dynamic process, and the category may change at any time. It must, therefore, be repeated at every stage of the evacuation chain. The expectant category refers to those critically injured casualties who will die despite the best care, and who will divert resources from those who can be salvaged. To do the most for the most means to leave the expectant patients to die, while those who are salvageable are treated.

18.10 (A) T (B) T (C) F (D) F (E) T

Amputation equipment need only be carried by a Mobile Surgical Team deployed specifically from hospital to perform a surgical procedure, then return to hospital with the patient. Resupply is generally from the ambulance equipment vehicle, with backup supplies coming from regional supply depots.

SHORT ANSWERS

18.11 The functions of the police at the scene are:

- Control of the incident
- Prevention of escalation of the incident
- Evacuation of those uninjured who are still in danger
- Ensuring the activation of other emergency services
- Provision of traffic control
- Liaison with and facilitation of other emergency services
- Maintenance of records of victims (survived, injured, died; and location)
- Identification of the dead
- Maintenance of public order
- Protection of property
- Criminal investigation
- Liaison with the media

18.12 Echo–November–Tango–Oscar–November–Oscar–Xray
Mike–Oscar–Romeo–Papa–Hotel–India–November–Echo
Kilo–Echo–Tango–Alpha–Mike–India–November–Echo

18.13 The following is a schematic diagram of a Casualty Clearing Station:

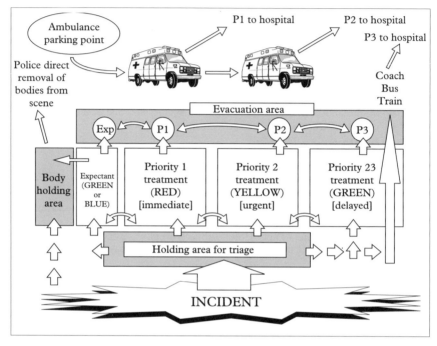

Adapted from Hodgetts, McNeil and Cooke, *The Pre-hospital Emergency Management Master.* BMJ Publications, London, 1995.

18.14 The *triage sieve* is a rapid 'first-look' triage and takes account of the patient's mobility and an assessment of their airway, breathing and circulation. It will generally take about 30 seconds to perform. The *triage sort* is a more detailed physiological assessment, based on the Triage Revised Trauma Score, and requires the respiratory rate, systolic blood pressure and Glasgow Coma Scale to be measured. The triage sort score ranges from 0 to 12, and this is used to assign a conventional triage priority. Priorities can be upgraded by the anatomical injury, if the current physiological status does not reflect the urgency for treatment (for example, a severed hand treated immediately by direct pressure and elevation may produce no significant change in the physiology, but requires 'urgent' rather than 'delayed' treatment).

PICTURE QUIZ

18.15 The priorities of the first ambulance crew on scene can be summarized as:

- *Command*
- *Safety* (self, scene, casualties: the 1-2-3 of safety)
- *Communication* (with control, using the ETHANE mnemonic)
- *Assessment* (to establish the number and severity of casualties, and the resources required immediately)

18.16 The commonly used triage priorities (civilian and military) are shown in the table below:

Treatment	Priority	Colour	Description
T1	P1	Red	Immediate
T2	P2	Yellow	Urgent
T3	P3	Green	Delayed
T4	P1 hold	Blue/other	Expectant
Dead	Dead	White/Black	Dead

The 'expectant' priority can be represented in a number of ways:

- Some card systems have a separate blue label
- On a cruciform folding card the 'ears' of the green label can be folded back to reveal the red label underneath
- 'Expectant' can be written across any colour of label
- The yellow label can be used: after all, you will treat the expectant when all the red have been treated!

In the end it does not matter what system is used: so long as everyone understands it.

CASE HISTORY

These four casualties have been assessed using the *triage sieve*.

Remember: TRIAGE SIEVE
1. Walking = GREEN
2. Not walking – assess breathing
3. No breathing and fails to breathe on opening airway = WHITE
4. Breathing, or starts to breathe on opening airway – count rate.
5. Respiratory rate <10 or >30 per minute = RED
6. Respiratory rate 10–30 per minute – assess circulation
7. Pulse >120 per minute or capillary refill >2 seconds = RED
8. Pulse <120 per minute or capillary refill <2 seconds = YELLOW

- If a patient can walk, the triage sieve says GREEN.
- No breathing and no pulse is DEAD in a major incident, and does not warrant resuscitation.
- A respiratory rate of less than 10 (or more than 30) is a breathing problem, and warrants a RED label. If the rate was between 10 and 30 per minute, the casualty would be RED on circulation grounds, as the pulse is >120 per minute. If the expectant category was instituted, this patient would be expectant.
- Normal respiratory rate, but abnormal circulation (pulse >120 per minute) requires a RED label.

MASS GATHERING AND SPORTS MEDICINE

Refer to Chapters 44 and 57 of *Emergency Care: A Textbook for Paramedics.*

MULTIPLE CHOICE

19.1 **The following are statutory equipment requirements to be available at the side of the pitch for a Premier League football match:**

A. Defibrillator

B. Long spinal board with head-box

C. Femoral traction splint

D. Cardiac arrest drugs

E. Kendrick extrication device

19.2 **The following are statutory requirements for resuscitation equipment for the public at an international airport:**

A. Defibrillator (semi-automatic)

B. Laerdal pocket mask

C. Bag-valve-mask device

D. Oxygen with flow meter

E. Portable suction

19.3 The following are the minimum statutory requirements for first aiders at a stadium event:

A. 1:1000 public

B. 1:2000 public

C. 1:500 public

D. 1:5000 public

E. 1:10,000 public

19.4 The following are the minimum statutory requirements for crowd doctors at a stadium event exceeding 2000 public:

A. 1:event

B. 1:2000 public

C. 1:5000 public

D. 1:10,000 public

E. None

19.5 The following are the minimum statutory requirements for nurses at a stadium event:

A. 2:event

B. 1:2000 public

C. 1:5000 public

D. 1:10,000 public

E. None

19.6 The following are recognized minimum training standards for first aiders at a stadium event:

A. Current St John first aid certificate

B. Current St Andrew first aid certificate

C. Current Red Cross first aid certificate

D. No formal training required

E. Scouting first aid certificate

19.7 **The following sports are associated with spinal injuries:**

A.   Rugby (scrum collapse)

B.   Horse riding

C.   Diving

D.   Motorsport

E.   Parachuting

SHORT ANSWERS

19.8 **Write short notes on the Taylor and Gibson reports.**

19.9 **You are asked to arrange the ambulance cover for an organized rave in a sports stadium, with an estimated 5000 crowd. What personnel and equipment do you think is essential?**

PICTURE QUIZ

19.10 **What injuries would you anticipate?**

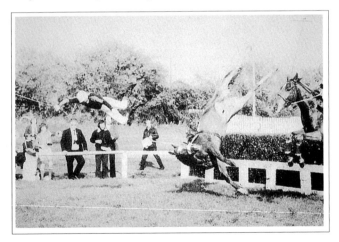

19.11 **What is the danger here?**

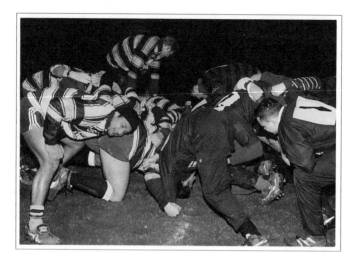

MASS GATHERING AND SPORTS MEDICINE

MULTIPLE CHOICE

19.1 **(A) T (B) F (C) F (D) F (E) F**

The only absolute medical equipment requirement for a Premier League football match is a defibrillator. However, most football clubs recognize the obligation to provide medical cover for their players (a player's doctor, or physiotherapist) and for the tens of thousands of fans (a crowd doctor and first aiders). First aid facilities and equipment are variable nationally, but go so far as to include a hospital with fully staffed and equipped resuscitation room and mobile X-ray unit plus multiple first aid units with advanced life support equipment at Wembley Stadium.

19.2 **(A) F (B) F (C) F (D) F (E) F**

There is no statutory requirement to provide a resuscitation facility for the public at an international airport. Airline companies provide a variable amount of equipment and drugs for use on domestic and international flights. A small number of companies (two at the time of press) provide a semi-automatic defibrillator on international flights. The drugs are generally intended for use by a doctor, who may be serendipitously on the flight.

19.3 **(A) T (B) F (C) F (D) F (E) F**

One first aider per 1000 public is required. This means that the larger Premier League clubs may have to provide 70–80 first aid trained staff for each match. Strategies to accommodate this include training the stewards, using uniformed St John staff, or employing personnel with a recognized first aid certificate (see question 19.6).

19.4 (A) T (B) F (C) F (D) F (E) F

Following the Taylor and Gibson reports (see answer 19.8) a minimum of one crowd doctor is recommended at any football match where the crowd exceeds 2000. This crowd doctor should be 'trained', and recognized training has included the Football Association's *Crowd Doctors' Course*, the *Pre-Hospital Emergency Care Certificate* (Royal College of Surgeons of Edinburgh) and the *Diploma in Immediate Medical Care* (Royal College of Surgeons of Edinburgh). Although on site to assist in treatment with medical emergencies within the crowd, this doctor will become the Medical Incident Officer in the event of a major incident. Separate major incident training is, therefore, important, such as the three day *MIMMS* (*Major Incident Medical Management and Support*) course.

19.5 (A) F (B) F (C) F (D) F (E) T

There is no statutory requirement for nurses to be present at a stadium event. Nurses are often employed, however, as first aiders or as stewards providing first aid, or in an official nursing role within first aid posts (and the hospital at Wembley) of the larger stadia.

19.6 (A) T (B) T (C) T (D) F (E) F

St Andrew is equivalent to the St John voluntary ambulance service organization in Scotland.

19.7 (A) T (B) T (C) T (D) T (E) T

An accident in any of these sports constitutes a risk of spinal injury. In rugby a scrum collapse is notorious for producing a cervical spine injury. In horse riding there is a fall from a significant height, perhaps compounded by the horse falling on top of the rider. In board diving there may be a hyperflexion injury if the head hits the bottom of the pool. This means there is an associated head injury and, if there is concussion, the victim may drown. *Always consider an associated spinal injury when rescuing a drowned victim in a pool or river.* In motorsport there will be rapid deceleration and blunt impact, with the risk of a 'whiplash' spinal injury. Parachuting is particularly associated with vertebral wedge (compression) fractures.

SHORT ANSWERS

19.8 Following the Hillsborough football stadium disaster on 15 April 1989 (95 killed, 200 injured) Lord Justice Taylor was commissioned to report on this incident and make recommendations to reduce the likelihood of a future event and to improve the response should such an event recur.* One outcome is the implementation of all seater stadia. The recommendations from this report for medical facilities were:

- One trained first aider per 1000 public
- One doctor present when the crowd is more than 2000, 'trained and competent in advanced first aid . . . and present one hour before kick off . . . and remain for half an hour after the end of the match'
- At least one fully equipped ambulance in attendance when the crowd exceeds 5000
- A major incident equipment vehicle capable of dealing with 50 casualties when there is a crowd exceeding 25,000
- A variable number of ambulances determined by the ambulance service in consultation with the local authority for crowds over 5000

Mr Myles Gibson was commissioned to prepare a subsidiary report on the medical requirements for a football match, and the recommendations confirm those of the Taylor report.

*Lord Justice Taylor. The Hillsborough Stadium Disaster: final report. HMSO 1990, London.

19.9 It is first necessary to consider the risk at such an event. Potential problems include:

- Drug-related illness (alcohol, Ecstasy, and others)
- Assault
- Medical problems (faint, fit, asthma)

The most likely serious adverse event would be related to drug toxicity, with a heat exhaustion picture secondary to Ecstasy. A variety of drugs are also sold to the unsuspecting youth to counter the side effects of stimulant drugs (e.g. beta-blockers to reduce tachycardia), which will complicate the management. For these reasons it may be appropriate to deploy a paramedic ambulance crew who have advanced circulation (infusion) and advanced cardiac life support skills.

PICTURE QUIZ

19.10 Injuries from falling off a horse are often serious and the following must be anticipated:

- Head injury
- Spinal injury
- Pelvic fracture
- Long bone fracture/major joint dislocation

If the horse rolls over the rider also consider:

- Rib fractures and pulmonary contusion/haemopneumothorax
- Abdominal visceral injury

If the horse stands on the rider also consider:

- Flail chest

19.11 The principal danger is a cervical spine injury on collapse of the scrum.

ADMINISTRATION, ETHICS AND THE LAW

Refer to Chapters 58, 59, 60, and Appendix D of *Emergency Care: A Textbook for Paramedics.*

20.1   The following are indications to discontinue resuscitation:

A.   Rescuer fatigue

B.   Ventricular fibrillation unresponsive to 12 DC shocks

C.   Fixed and dilated pupils

D.   Agonal rhythm

E.   An obstructed upper airway that cannot be relieved by back blows and abdominal thrusts

20.2   The following are indications not to start resuscitation:

A.   Heavy chemical contamination

B.   Rigor mortis

C.   Age over 90 years

D.   Hypothermia below 30°C

E.   Drowning for more than 30 minutes

20.3   If a doctor and a paramedic are present at the scene, the following are the ethical or statutory responsibilities of the doctor:

A.   To supervise all patient care at the scene

B.   To determine the best mode of transport from the scene

C.   To determine the patient care during transport

D.   To alert the hospital

E.   To pronounce death

20.4 The components of the Triage Revised Trauma Score include:

A. Respiratory rate

B. Capillary refill time

C. Respiratory effort

D. Glasgow Coma Scale

E. Systolic and diastolic blood pressure

20.5 Negligence requires the following to be proven:

A. A duty of care

B. A failure to perform in a manner equivalent to one's peers

C. A failure to perform according to the opinion of an independent expert

D. Deliberate harm to the patient

E. A deleterious effect on the patient

20.6 You are about to start resuscitation when the patient's spouse shows you a living will requesting no active resuscitation. The following actions are appropriate:

A. Start resuscitation and continue to hospital

B. Immediately stop resuscitation

C. Start resuscitation while you assess the situation

D. Discontinue resuscitation when immediately treatable causes have been identified

E. None of the above

20.7 Concerning medical audit:

A. A principal aim is to identify an individual officer's mistakes

B. Its main intention is to improve patient care

C. It involves measuring performance against an agreed standard

D. It means the same as medical research

E. It cannot be done at station level

CASE HISTORY 1

An elderly man with known advanced carcinoma of the lung has taken 30 codydramol tablets, which contain a lethal dose of opiate and a lethal dose of paracetamol. His respiratory rate is 4 per minute on your arrival, and he stops breathing shortly after. What would you do?

CASE HISTORY 2

You attend an adult who has fallen 7 metres and sustained a serious head injury. The Glasgow Coma Scale is 3 and there is some blood in the upper airway. You attempt intubation, but place the tube in the oesophagus. This is recognized and, after a period of reoxygenation, intubation is attempted for the second time, again unsuccessfully. At this stage you decide to insert an oropharyngeal airway, ventilate the patient with a bag-valve-mask device and provide suction, while moving to hospital. Have you been negligent in failing to secure the airway by intubation?

ADMINISTRATION, ETHICS AND THE LAW

MULTIPLE CHOICE

20.1   (A) T (B) F (C) F (D) T (E) F

After 12 shocks in ventricular fibrillation, sodium bicarbonate, lignocaine or bretylium are recommended. Fixed pupils are not a reliable sign of death, particularly when a mydriatic drug (pupil dilating, such as atropine) has been given.

An obstructed airway that cannot be relieved by back blows and abdominal thrusts requires, if a foreign body cannot be removed with a laryngoscope and Magill's forceps, the obstruction to be bypassed by a needle or surgical cricothyrotomy.

20.2   (A) T (B) T (C) F (D) F (E) T

If adequate personal protective clothing is not available, then a heavily contaminated chemical casualty should not be treated. Age alone is not an indicator to withold resuscitation, but if a patient has been immersed for more than 30 minutes resuscitation is unlikely to be successful (with the possible exception of a child immersed in freezing water).

20.3   (A) T (B) F (C) T (D) F (E) T

It is an ambulance service responsibility to determine the best way to transport a patient to hospital, although the doctor would have a responsibility to advise on what treatment is appropriate during the journey.

Some ambulance services provide a protocol that allows their paramedics to pronounce death. In general, it would be the responsibiity of a doctor to pronounce death if one were present at the scene.

20.4 (A) T (B) F (C) F (D) T (E) F

The *Triage Revised Trauma Score* is a tool designed by Howard Champion (trauma surgeon, Washington DC) to assist paramedics in the United States in deciding whether to transport a trauma victim to the nearest hospital or to a Trauma Center. It is a physiological score with three elements:

- Glasgow Coma Scale
- Systolic blood pressure
- Respiratory rate

Each of these is scored from 0 to 4, and a fall in one point in any parameter is an indication to transport directly to the Trauma Center.

The *Trauma Score* originally developed by Champion in 1981 also included the capillary refill time and 'respiratory effort' (maximum score 16), but both of these were found to be unreliable in the field. The *Revised Trauma Score* uses the same scoring system as the TRTS, but multiplies each parameter by a weighting coefficient which reflects the relative importance of each vital sign. This is a retrospective audit tool.

20.5 (A) T (B) T (C) F (D) F (E) T

For negligence to be proven, three factors need to be satisfied:

- There must have been a duty of care to that patient
- There must have been a failure to execute the duty of care
- The patient must have suffered in some way as a result of the failure to execute the duty of care

20.6 (A) T (B) T (C) F (D) F (E) F

In the majority of ambulance services, a paramedic does not have the privilege of pronouncing death after resuscitation is started. Once begun, therefore, the paramedic is generally obliged to continue until the patient is transported to hospital.

Common sense and protocol will dictate clear circumstances where to start resuscitation is inappropriate, such as decapitation, or the presence of rigor mortis.

This situation is extremely difficult, and there may be no absolutely correct answer, but two options are defensible:

- To respect the living will in a patient who has no vital signs and not to attempt resuscitation
- To ignore the living will if it is thought there is a chance of survival by instituting resuscitation and continuing this to hospital

The incidence of living wills is likely to increase with time.

20.7   (A) F (B) T (C) T (D) F (E) F

The aim of medical audit is to improve patient care and the clinical audit process is based on the following logical sequence of events:

1. Identify a problem area in patient management
2. Establish a standard of care for that problem area
3. Measure performance against that agreed standard
4. Analyse the results and identify areas for improvement
5. Educate staff
6. Implement the necessary changes to the clinical pathway
7. Remeasure the performance against the original standard to confirm improvement
8. Establish new and higher standards, and restart the process

Research in general involves a direct comparison of two or more methods of managing a problem area to determine the best approach.

Audit can be undertaken at any level, and could certainly be performed at station level.

CASE HISTORY 1

The potential dilemma in this case is to decide whether or not to start resuscitation with the history of carcinoma.

The paramedic is at a disadvantage, as it is unlikely that he or she will be familiar with the patient's past history and what is said by a relative will have to be taken at face value without substantiation.

Additionally, the effects of this overdose are reversible: the respiratory depression from the opiate is reversible with naloxone, and the paracetamol toxicity is reversible with *N*-acetyl cysteine administered in hospital.

In this case, the most appropriate solution is probably to support the airway and breathing and administer naloxone (if carried), then transport to hospital for further treatment.

CASE HISTORY 2

It is not negligent to intubate the oesophagus, only to fail to recognize this has occurred and to take the appropriate remedial steps. You have not failed in your duty of care if an endotracheal tube cannot be passed. In general, *it is not a lack of intubation that kills, but a lack of oxygenation.* When an advanced airway manoeuvre fails, it would be appropriate to return to more basic airway manoeuvres such as bag-valve-mask with an airway adjunct. In this respect the paramedic should be complemented, not chastised, on their actions which could be considered as 'textbook'.

MULTIPLE CHOICE

TP.1   With complete heart block:

A.   There are more Ps than QRSs on a rhythm strip

B.   The ventricular rate is regular

C.   Pre-hospital treatment usually includes external pacing

D.   The patient may give a history of fainting

E.   Adrenaline will speed up the ventricular rate

TP.2   A motorcyclist has hit a car and has a suspected unstable fracture of the pelvis and a closed fracture of the right femur. The following are true:

A.   Leather trousers should be cut to examine the right thigh

B.   A Sager-type traction splint should be applied

C.   The patient is at risk from life-threatening haemorrhage

D.   A cervical collar should always be applied

E.   Supplemental oxygen is required only if the saturation is reduced on the pulse oximeter

TP.3   Concerning pre-hospital analgesia:

A.   Nalbuphine is contraindicated following abdominal injury

B.   Entonox provides equivalent analgesia to 10 mg morphine IV

C.   Pain will exacerbate the physiological effects of shock

D.   Splintage is part of pre-hospital pain relief

E.   Entonox is contraindicated when surgical emphysema is present

TP.4 The following are true of a major incident:

A. A major incident is any incident involving more than 25 casualties

B. A compound incident is one where the lines of communication or transportation are disrupted

C. The officer in overall control at a major incident is the most senior ranked officer present, irrespective of service

D. Communication is the commonest failing

E. The first ambulance crew on scene must triage and treat the most severely injured

TP.5 A 55-year-old man with a history of angina dials 999 after 45 minutes of central chest pain, unrelieved by GTN (glyceryl trinitrate):

A. It should be assumed that the patient has suffered a myocardial infarction

B. Aspirin must be given

C. GTN can be repeated

D. Oxygen should be administered at ~4 L/min

E. The diagnosis may be oesophageal spasm

TP.6 The following are true of children:

A. They are more prone to hypothermia than adults

B. Hypoglycaemia is a common complication of severe illness

C. The palm of a child's hand represents 1% of its body surface area

D. Weight (in kilograms) can be estimated from the formula [age + 2] × 4

E. Trauma is the second commonest cause of death in children aged 1–15 years

TP.7 Concerning meningococcal meningitis:

A. A purpuric rash strongly suggests meningococcal meningitis

B. Penicillin given by the general practitioner will improve the outcome

C. The ambulance crew always requires antibiotics to prevent infection

D. This is the least common bacterial meningitis in children

E. Onset of symptoms to death is often less than 12 hours

TP.8 **The following are typical features of a tricyclic antidepressant overdose:**

A. Pinpoint pupils

B. Aggressive and excitable behaviour

C. Tachycardia

D. Associated alcohol intoxication

E. Fitting

TP.9 **At the scene of a bomb:**

A. Radios should not be used until declared safe to do so by the police

B. The Army Bomb Disposal Unit are in overall control

C. The safe distance from an unexploded device is 200 metres

D. Blast lung is a common complication of survivors

E. Most injuries will result from fragmentation

TP.10 **The following are components of the Triage Revised Trauma Score:**

A. Systolic blood pressure

B. Capillary refill time

C. Pulse rate

D. Glasgow Coma Scale

E. Respiratory rate

SHORT ANSWERS

TP.11 You are the first emergency vehicle to arrive at the scene of a road accident where an elderly driver has hit four pedestrians at a bus stop. The car has ploughed into a wall. The driver is trapped, and one pedestrian is under the car. How would you structure a radio message to Ambulance Control?

TP.12 What are the key differences in the basic life support protocols for an adult and an infant (<1 year)?

PICTURE QUIZ

TP.13 This teenager was trapped by his arm in a factory machine for 40 minutes.

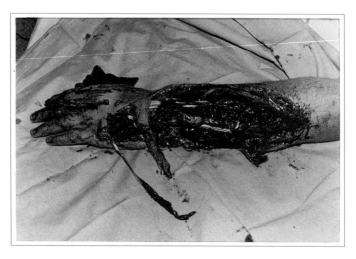

- What are the priorities of management?
- What analgesic techniques could be used to effect a release?

CASE HISTORY

A 5-year-old boy has fallen through the ice over a canal on a December morning. Twenty minutes after the boy fell through the ice, the Fire Service rescue the child who is pale, floppy and not breathing. You can feel no pulse and the cardiac monitor shows asystole.

- What do you do?
- What factors would help you to determine whether or not to resuscitate?

MULTIPLE CHOICE

TP.1   (A) T (B) T (C) F (D) T (E) T

First-degree heart block is simply a prolongation of the PR interval. With second- or third-degree heart block there is incomplete or absent transmission of impulses from the atria to the ventricles. There are, therefore, more P waves than QRS complexes on the ECG rhythm strip.

In third-degree block the P-wave (atrial) rate is regular and the QRS (ventricular) rate is regular, but the rates are different so that the PR interval is variable.

External pacing systems are not used by the ambulance services in the UK, although they may be used by immediate care doctors.

TP.2   (A) F (B) F (C) T (D) T (E) F

A motorcyclist's tight leather trousers may splint the pelvis, and on release of this garment there may be an increase in bleeding from an unstable fractured pelvis. Additionally, the secondary survey at the scene is limited by time and any unnecessary exposure to the elements. Nothing would be gained by exposing a closed fracture of the femur at the scene.

Traction splints are contraindicated with unstable pelvic fractures because the countertraction is exerted against the pelvis.

A significant force is required to fracture the pelvis or femur. When this is the result of generalized blunt trauma, such as a road traffic accident, it must be assumed that the cervical spine has been injured until proven otherwise by X-ray and examination at hospital. It would be correct to immobilize this patient with a semi-rigid collar plus a head-box and spinal board.

All victims of significant trauma require supplemental high-concentration oxygen, irrespective of their saturation reading on a pulse oximeter.

TP.3   (A) F (B) T (C) T (D) T (E) T

Nalbuphine is a synthetic morphine-like drug, but weaker in action. Surgeons have stated that morphine given to a patient with abdominal pain before clinical examination may mask the clinical signs. *This is not an adequate reason to withold analgesia from a patient in severe pain.*

Entonox (50% oxygen + 50% nitrous oxide) is a powerful analgesic, equivalent to ~10 mg morphine IV. Scepticism of its effectiveness is often related to a failure to administer it correctly. The gas should be inhaled for about 2–3 minutes before any procedure (such as a manipulation or extrication) is attempted.

Entonox is contraindicated when there is any evidence of pneumothorax (including surgical emphysema) as the nitrous oxide will diffuse rapidly into the pneumothorax and cause it to tension.

Shock (inadequate tissue perfusion) results in the release of adrenaline which causes peripheral vasoconstriction and a tachycardia. Pain produces a similar physiological response, and as such it will exacerbate the physiological effects of shock.

TP.4 (A) F (B) T (C) F (D) T (E) F

A major incident for the health services requires extraordinary resources: 25 casualties with minor injuries in an urban environment can be coped with by normal resources. The definition cannot, therefore, be solely a reflection of the number of casualties.

Major incidents are subclasssified as follows:

- Natural (e.g. earthquake) or man-made
- Simple or compound (communication/transportation disrupted)
- Compensated or uncompensated (no amount of resources allows coping)

The officer in control is the senior *Police* officer, unlike the armed services where it is the most senior ranking officer irrespective of service.

The responsibilities of the first ambulance crew on scene are:

- To command subsequent ambulance resources until relieved by the designated Ambulance Incident Officer
- To ensure safety of themselves, the scene and the casualties
- To assess the scene for the number and severity of casualties, and the initial ambulance and medical response required
- To communicate with control

They must *not* become involved with triage, treatment or transport of casualties.

TP.5   (A) T (B) F (C) T (D) F (E) T

Central chest pain unrelieved by GTN that lasts more than 20 minutes should be assumed to be a myocardial infarction. In the context of a patient with known ischaemic heart disease, it is the most likely diagnosis, but other potential diagnoses will include:

- Dissecting thoracic aortic aneurysm
- Oesophageal spasm
- Pancreatitis
- Perforated duodenal ulcer

Aspirin will reduce the mortality following a myocardial infarction, but its timing is not critical (needs to be given within the first 24 hours) and as such it is not essential that it is administered as soon as the diagnosis is made.

High-concentration oxygen should be given, at a flow rate of 10–15 L/minute.

TP.6   (A) T (B) T (C) T (D) F (E) F

Children have a larger surface area to volume ratio than adults and will cool more rapidly when exposed. Children also have limited liver glycogen stores, and when 'stressed' by illness or injury will utilize these stores rapidly, after which time they may become hypoglycaemic.

The formula to estimate a child's weight between 1 and 10 years is:

$$\text{Weight (kg)} = [\text{age (years)} + 4] \times 2$$

Trauma is the commonest cause of death from 1 to 15 years.

TP.7   (A) F (B) T (C) F (D) F (E) T

Meningococcal meningitis is the most virulent form of bacterial meningitis. The time from onset of symptoms, which may be mistaken for influenza, and death is frighteningly short and often less than 12 hours.

A purpuric rash (bleeding under the skin, so rash does not blanch) indicates meningococcal septicaemia, *not* meningococcal meningitis. Septicaemia is much less common, but it has a worse prognosis: deaths are usually a result of hypovolaemic shock.

Prophylactic antibiotics are *not* required by the ambulance crew unless mouth to mouth ventilation has been given (only so-called 'kissing contacts' need antibiotics).

The relative importance of meningococcal meningitis has increased since 1992 when the *Haemophilus influenza* (Hib) vaccination was introduced.

TP.8   (A) F (B) F (C) T (D) T (E) T

Tricyclic antidepressant overdose is relatively common. The pupils will be dilated, and pinpoint pupils would suggest an opiate overdose. Patients will usually have a depressed level of consciousness or be comatose, not excitable. Convulsions may occur.

Sinus tachycardia is the most consistent ECG abnormality, although any tachydysrhythmia may be seen. If there is no sinus tachycardia, there is unlikely to be any significant tricyclic poisoning.

Alcohol is often taken in association with *any* overdose of tablets.

TP.9   (A) T (B) F (C) F (D) F (E) T

Secondary devices are common at the scene of a bomb, and these may be radio controlled. Radios should not be used until it has been declared safe to do so by the police. It is the civilian police, not the Army Bomb Disposal Unit, who are in overall control at the scene of a bomb.

The safe distance from an unexploded device is 600 metres.

Blast lung is rare in survivors close to the point of explosion (less than 1% of survivors), but it would be suspected if the patient is short of breath or gives other symptoms of exposure to a significant blast load (such as deafness from perforated ear drums).

The vast majority of injuries following an explosion will be the result of fragmentation. Fragments are described as *primary* if they come from the bomb itself, or *secondary* if they are debris carried by the blast wind. Other mechanisms of injury are the blast wave, the blast wind, crush from falling masonry, flash burns and psychological trauma.

TP.10   (A) T (B) F (C) F (D) T (E) T

The *Triage Revised Trauma Score* was designed to assist paramedics in the United States in deciding whether to take a patient directly to a Trauma Center, or to the nearest hospital. Three physiological variables are scored from 0 to 4:

- Systolic blood pressure
- Glasgow Coma Scale
- Respiratory rate

The scores are added together and, if there is a fall by one point in any parameter (total score less than or equal to 11), there is an increased likelihood of death necessitating direct transport to a Trauma Center.

The original Trauma Score also included capillary refill time and 'respiratory effort', neither of which could be reliably measured in the field.

SHORT ANSWERS

TP.11 The radio message to Ambulance Control can be structured by using the mnemonic *ETHANE:*

E	Exact location
T	Type of incident (RTA, car hit pedestrians)
H	Hazards, present and potential (petrol? fire?)
A	Access to the scene (has traffic blocked one carriageway?)
N	Number and severity of casualties (5 casualties; 2 persons trapped)
E	Emergency services present and required (require 2 ambulances, police, and fire and rescue)

TP.12 The principal differences in the basic life support protocols are shown in the table below.

Infant	Adult
Shake and shout	
• May cry, open eyes or startle	• May open eyes and talk
Airway	
• Do not overextend head	• Fully extend head
• No blind finger sweep	• Finger sweep OK
Breathing	
• If not breathing give 5 breaths	• If not breathing give 2 breaths
Circulation	
• Check brachial pulse	• Check carotid pulse
• Use 2 fingers for chest compressions	• Use 2 hands for chest compressions
• Compress 1 finger's breadth below internipple line	• Compress 2 finger's breadth above xiphisternum
Help	
• Go for help after 20 cycles 5:1 compressions:ventilations	• Go for help after 2 ventilations

PICTURE QUIZ

TP.13 The priorities for management are:

- Scene safety: prevent others being injured and further injury to the casualty
- *Airway:* open, clear and secure
- *Breathing:* give high-flow oxygen, check for life-threatening injuries
- *Circulation:* stop external bleeding by direct pressure and elevation, set up an intravenous infusion

Communicate the details to the hospital so the Trauma Team is on standby to receive the casualty.

Analgesic options to facilitate release from the machinery are:

- Entonox (in this case it was inadequate)
- Nalbuphine (in this case it was inadequate)
- Morphine by a doctor (but nalbuphine given will inhibit the action of morphine as it is a *partial antagonist*)
- Ketamine by a doctor (this was given and was highly effective)
- General anaesthetic by a doctor (this was not required in this case)

CASE HISTORY

This child is clinically dead. However, survival without neurological compromise is documented in victims of cold water drowning with prolonged submersion.

In this instance, the appropriate action is to start basic life support and move rapidly to hospital where advanced cardiac life support including aggressive active rewarming should take place. Ventricular fibrillation is unlikely to be responsive to defibrillation when the core temperature is below 30°C.

The decision whether to start resuscitation can be difficult, but if in doubt start resuscitation and leave the decision to discontinue to the hospital Accident and Emergency senior doctor. There are no absolute rules. Factors that may influence your decision in this case history situation are:

- Age of the patient (lower threshold for starting resuscitation in children)
- Temperature of the water (rapid cooling effect may favourably influence resuscitation)
- Length of time in the water (over one hour will make the decision more difficult)

Index

Numbers in italic refer to tables or illustrations; numbers in bold refer to main discussion.

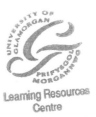